AN HISTORICAL ACCOUNT OF PHARMACOLOGY TO THE 20TH CENTURY

Publication Number 970
AMERICAN LECTURE SERIES®

A Publication in
The BANNERSTONE DIVISION *of*
AMERICAN LECTURES IN PHARMACOLOGY

Editor
DOCTOR ELTON L. McCAWLEY
Department of Pharmacology
University of Oregon Medical School
Portland, Oregon

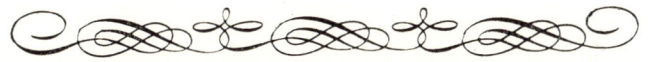

AN HISTORICAL ACCOUNT OF PHARMACOLOGY
TO THE 20th CENTURY

By

CHAUNCEY D. LEAKE
*University of California
San Francisco*

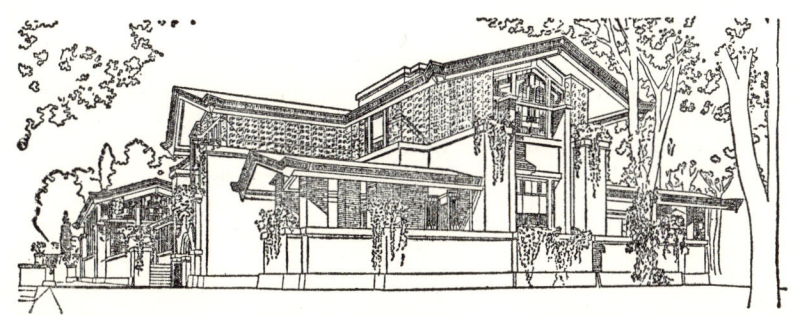

CHARLES C THOMAS • PUBLISHER
Springfield • Illinois • U.S.A.

Published and Distributed Throughout the World by
CHARLES C THOMAS • PUBLISHER
BANNERSTONE HOUSE
301-327 East Lawrence Avenue, Springfield, Illinois, U.S.A.

This book is protected by copyright. No part of it may be reproduced in any manner without written permission from the publisher.

© *1975, by* CHARLES C THOMAS • PUBLISHER
ISBN 0-398-03277-7 cloth
0-398-03278-5 paper
Library of Congress Catalog Card Number: 74-13219

With THOMAS BOOKS *careful attention is given to all details of manufacturing and design. It is the Publisher's desire to present books that are satisfactory as to their physical qualities and artistic possibilities and appropriate for their particular use.* THOMAS BOOKS *will be true to those laws of quality that assure a good name and good will.*

Printed in the United States of America
N-1

Library of Congress Cataloging in Publication Data

Leake, Chauncey Depew, 1896-
   An historical account of pharmacology.

   (American lecture series, publication no. 970. A monograph in the Bannerstone Division of American lectures in pharmacology)
   1. Pharmacology—History   I. Title.
[DNLM: 1. Drugs—History. 2. Pharmacology—History. QV11 L435h]
RM41.L4   615′.1′09   74-13219
ISBN 0-398-03277-7
ISBN 0-398-03278-5 (pbk.)

This book, on which I've worked for so long, is dedicated with deep affection to all who have struggled with me in the twisting coils of pharmacology and toxicology, from Elizabeth, my wife, to the hundreds of colleagues and students who have added so much to what I've tried to do.

> To hundreds who have toiled along
> with me, who was "Old Man"
> for many years in warm
> companionship, I often can
> return in pleasant thought
> and see again the busy place,
> and hear ideas take form,
> as information flowed apace.
>
> We found a lasting joy in work
> we did together; when we went
> away, we held our precious bond,
> and kept our pride of time well spent.
> So others carry on where we
> leave off: may they as joyful be!

CHAUNCEY LEAKE

Look at the names—long complex chemical names, with methyls and hydroxies and pyrimidyls, and say it's much too complicated. Well, it is complicated. But automobiles are complicated, too, and so are television transmitters and flying clippers and sub-machine guns and synthetic silk stockings and all the other triumphs of our day. They're just as complicated as they can be—and yet we use them because they give the results we want. In the very same way, we use pure drugs against disease or let a doctor use them on us; for to most of us it's the result that counts and not the complex reason behind it.

MILTON SILVERMAN (1941)
Magic in a Bottle

PREFACE

THIS BOOK HAS BEEN AN enjoyable task. I've learned much. It has been a difficult job, however, complicated by inhibitory advice, by lack of secretarial aid, and by the pressure of many responsibilities. Every effort had been made to have this book on hand for the 5th International Congress of Pharmacology, to be held in San Francisco in July, 1972. But this was not to be!

This book is not conventional. There is no critical apparatus, not a complicating footnote, and no argumentative detail. References are given directly in the text. They are, I think, sufficient to indicate the sources of my information, and thus of my opinions. As one reads along, one may readily learn to skip them if one wishes to do so.

I make no pretence at snobbish scholarship. Having spent many years in pharmacology laboratories, especially at the University of Wisconsin and the University of California in San Francisco, I think that I am reasonably familiar with the joys and sorrows of discovering biomedical factual and verifiable data by direct experimentation on animals and humans, including myself. For over fifty years I have taught pharmacology in various ways, but always with an historical orientation. Thus, my ideas, as offered in this book, have long been tested, modified, and often reversed.

It disappoints me to realize that when I think I have so much of pharmacology to share with others, I am asked so seldom to do so. This is one of the penalties of age. Thus I take comfort and pleasure in writing this book, in the hope that an occasional reader may find inspiration and stimulus from the often confusing but rarely tiresome story of the acquisition of the monumental amount of pharmacological information we now have. What will we do with it all? Here is the challenge to the best of our imaginative skill, hopefully directed toward the benefit of all life in what really could be the joy of living.

This book, I realize, does not tell a simple coherent story. Pharmacology is too complex a subject for that. My often disjointed historical account of the development of drugs is thus more of a chronological compendium than a smoothly flowing history. It has thus required much care on my part to be as accurate as I can be on facts, and as reasonable as possible on interpretative discussion. Mistakes aplenty will be found in this book; more, I fear, of omission than of commission.

My story of pharmacology and toxicology is more appropriate for intelligent people generally than it is for professional pharmacologists or professional historians of medicine or science. These professional historians and pharmacologists have their own conventional concepts and attitudes, with which I am not always in sympathy. Let me talk then as an amateur to fellow amateurs. If the professionals get anything from my presentation, they are welcome to it, of course. But I am not writing either for their praise or criticism, but rather for the amusement and possible interest of novices and amateurs who may wish to know something about the development of our knowledge about drugs.

I am grateful to Penny Lydecker for much aid in typing. An ever continuing source of encouragement in this and other ventures is my wife, Elizabeth. She has made helpful corrections and suggestions and has generally cheered me on. After half a century of pharmacology she could be forgiven for being fed up with it. She needs no forgiveness: she finds pharmacology more exciting than ever. So do I. We enjoy sharing our enthusiasms with others. Thus this book.

C.D.L.
The Upper Haight-Ashbury,
in San Francisco.

He preferred to know the power of herbs and their value for curing purposes, and, heedless of glory, to exercise that quiet art.

Virgil (70-19 BC)
Aenid, xii

OTHER BOOKS BY CHAUNCEY LEAKE

Percival's Medical Ethics, Williams & Wilkins, Baltimore, 1927

William Harvey's De Motu Cordis, annotated translation and commentary, CC Thomas, Springfield, Ill., 1928; 2nd edition, 1930; 3rd edition, 1941; 4th edition, 1957; 5th edition, 1970

The Opportunity for Pictorial Art in Modern Medicine: An Example in San Francisco, Privately printed, San Francisco, 1937

Travelogue 1938, Privately printed, San Francisco, 1938

California's Medical Story in Fresco, Privately printed, San Francisco, 1939

Allegory 1945, Privately printed, Galveston, 1945

Letheon: The Cadenced Story of Anesthesia, University of Texas Press, Austin, 1947

Can We Agree?, with Patrick Romanell, University of Texas Press, Austin, 1950

Ashbel Smith and Yellow Fever in Galveston, University of Texas Press, Austin, 1951

The Old Egyptian Medical Papyri, University of Kansas Press, Lawrence, 1952

Tissue Culture Cadences, Privately printed, Galveston, 1953

James Blake, M.D., On the Relation between Chemical Constitution and Biological Action, Indianapolis, 1955

Some Founders of Physiology, American Physiological Society, Washington, D.C., 1956

The Amphetamines, CC Thomas, Springfield, Ill., 1959

Alcoholic Beverages in Clinical Medicine, with Milton Silverman, Year Book Medical Publishers, Chicago, 1966

What Are We Living For? Practical Philosophy, Part 1: The Ethics, PJD Publications, Ltd., Westbury, New York, 1973

What Are We Living For? Practical Philosophy, Part 2: The Logics, PJD Publications, Ltd., Westbury, New York, 1974

CONTENTS

	Page
Dedication	v
Preface	vii

Chapter

1.	AN HISTORICAL ACCOUNT OF PHARMACOLOGY	3
2.	PROTOPHARMACOLOGY: PREHISTORIC EMPIRICAL DRUG LORE	17
3.	PROTOPHARMACOLOGY: CODIFIED EMPIRICAL DRUG USE	30
4.	GRAECO-ROMAN MEDICINE	57
5.	THE MUSLIM DRUG INNOVATIONS	71
6.	DRUGS IN MEDIEVAL EUROPE	82
7.	DRUG DEVELOPMENT IN THE RENAISSANCE	88
8.	DRUGS IN THE SEVENTEENTH AND EIGHTEENTH CENTURIES	101
9.	THE FIRST PART OF THE NINETEENTH CENTURY	119
10.	PHARMACOLOGY IN THE SECOND HALF OF THE NINETEENTH CENTURY	140
11.	PROGRESS AND PROMISE: TRANSITION OF PHARMACOLOGY FROM THE 19TH CENTURY INTO THE 20TH	170

Index	191

AN HISTORICAL ACCOUNT OF PHARMACOLOGY TO THE 20TH CENTURY

The physician without physiology and chemistry flounders along in an aimless fashion, never able to gain any accurate conception of disease, practicing a sort of popgun pharmacy, hitting now the malady and again the patient, he himself not knowing which.

WILLIAM OSLER (1849-1919)
Aequanimitas, 1900

CHAPTER 1

AN HISTORICAL ACCOUNT OF PHARMACOLOGY

Learn from the beasts the physic of the field,
ALEXANDER POPE (1688-1744)
An Essay on Man

INTRODUCTION

IN TRYING TO DEVELOP a coherent historical account of a subject, it is wise to indicate the limits of the discussion, that is, to define the subject. Pharmacology currently is considered to be the scientific discipline concerned with the interactions of chemical agents (drugs) and living material, whether or not the actions are good or bad for the living material, or whether the living material is plant or animal in origin. More broadly, pharmacology may be defined, as was done by the Viennese pharmacologists, Hans Horst Meyer (1853-1939) and Rudolph Gottlieb (1864-1924) in their classic text (1910), as the study of the effects of changes in the chemical environment of living material.

This definition of pharmacology has an advantage in suggesting that there may be both positive and negative feedback from chemical changes in living environments, and that the chemical environment of living material is dynamic. With current interest in the range of organizational levels of living material from macromolecules to ecologies, one may appreciate that pharmacology is, indeed, a big and busy subject.

The Greek-derived term, pharmacology, comes from *pharmakos,* a harmful item to be cast out, and *logos,* the word, or the truth about a matter, or as we say now, the study of something.

When one studies the harmful effects of drugs or chemicals on living things, one is concerned with toxicology, from the Greek word *toxikon,* a poison, or a poisoned arrow.

Practically, pharmacology and toxicology go together, for the harmful or poisonous or toxic effects of drugs are usually the result of quantitative extension, dose related, of the ordinary actions of the drugs. Distinctions between possible useful actions of drugs and their potentially toxic effects were recognized anciently. E. Harnack (1852-1915) gives many examples from classical sources of early appreciation of poisons and of toxic effects of drugs on humans in his *Das Gift in der Dramatischen und in der Antiken Litteratur* (Leipzig, F. Vogel, 1908, 78 pp.).

The borderline between pharmacology and toxicology is difficult to define. Many drugs produce allergic symptoms in susceptible people, and undesired side effects are apt to occur in the use of almost any drug. This problem of untoward drug action was first explored by Louis Lewin (1850-1929), the great Berlin toxicologist, in his *Die Nebenwirkungen der Arzneimittel* (Berlin, Hirschwald, 1881). The difficulty of unpredictable undesired side effects of drugs plagues the U.S. Food and Drug Administration in its effort to permit, in accordance with poorly drawn laws, only safe drugs to be marketed or prescribed. There are no absolutely safe drugs.

Lewin's historical study of poisons and poisoning is a classic *(Die Gifte in der Weltgeschichte,* Berlin, Springer, 1920), as is his *Die Pfeilgifte* (Leipzig, Barth, 1923). David I. Macht has given a fine account, with bibliography, of Louis Lewin (*Ann Med Hist,* n.s. *3:*179-194, 1931).

From its tentative beginnings, the study of drugs has been closely allied to therapeutics, and indeed, during the latter part of the nineteenth century and the early part of the twentieth it was customary for texts on the subject to be called *Pharmacology and Therapeutics.* Drug therapy of the sick and injured is merely one form of treatment; others, equally empirical at their beginning, are exercise, entertainment, bathing, massage, interviewing, and surgery. Drugs are now used in part in all forms of therapy. In surgery, for example, drugs are paramount in antisepsis, anesthesia, and in suppression of immune responses.

The union of pharmacology with therapeutics was natural enough when the whole endeavor of the health professions was directed solely to taking care of sick and injured people, of which there were plenty. In medical practice now, however, pharmacological knowledge can be applied to the (1) diagnosis of disease, (2) prevention of disease, (3) cure of disease, (4) alleviation of the symptoms of disease, and (5) promotion of optimum health. These strictly medical applications are made chiefly to individual people, and the emphasis here is on the person as a whole. Similarly, applications of pharmacology are made in dentistry, nursing, veterinary medicine, pharmacy, and in many of the health services, such as physical therapy, radiation technology, clinical laboratory technology, dietetics, and social service, and even in hospital administration and health insurance. Pharmacological knowledge is applied at a social level in public health and epidemiological control. Drugs are commanding much public attention and political interest in an effort to reduce their exploitation and to assure their relative safety and effectiveness. Further, applications of pharmacology are vigorously developing in agriculture, in agronomy in regulation of fertility and growth, in sociology in relation to drug abuse and addiction, in law, in environmental and pollution control, in economics and in international politics. Whenever chemicals are used on a large scale, as in agriculture or pest control, there is an ever-present possibility of toxic hazard. This can be deliberately exploited as in chemical warfare or riot control.

With scientific exploration of drug action on the one hand, and with social and environmental aspects of chemical use on the other hand, pharmacology and toxicology cover the range of organizational levels of living material from macromolecules through subcellular units, cells, organs and tissues, individuals and societies, to broad ecologies, or to global and space environments. It is a subject allied with, but quite distinct from and independent of biochemistry, physiology, pathology, microbiology, anatomy, and all aspects of individual and social disease. In the biomedical curriculum, pharmacology provides a natural bridge from the basic scientific disciplines to the practical clinical problems which beset us.

As I indicated in my presidential address before the American Association for the Advancement of Science in 1961, pharmacology as a science is concerned with certain problems involving the interactions of chemicals and living material which are unique to it and not usually considered by related sciences. These problems are (1) dose-effect and time-concentration relationships as analyzed by J. W. Trevan (1887-1955), and A. J. Clark (1885-1941); (2) the ways by which chemicals are absorbed and distributed in living material, the ways by which they are modified therein, and removed therefrom, as glimpsed by that brilliant Parisian, François Magendie (1783-1855) and as systematically developed by M. Von Nencki (1847-1911); (3) the localization of the site of interaction of chemicals and living material, as first fruitfully examined by Magendie's pupil, Claude Bernard (1813-1878), in showing that curare causes paralysis by blocking neuromuscular junctions; (4) the specific way by which chemicals and living material interact, again as first successfully explored by Claude Bernard in the case of carbon monoxide and hemoglobin, and (5) the relationship between the structure of a chemical agent and its biological activity, as first analyzed by James Blake (1814-1893), another pupil of Magendie, in regard to inorganic salts, and by T. R. Fraser (1841-1920) in respect to alkaloids.

The development of pharmacology as a broad and challenging scientific discipline has been long and varied. For centuries there was an empirical protopharmacology, with a slow and often erroneous effort to collect, analyze, codify and transmit information on crude drugs as gained by experience in various parts of the world. With the rise of quantitative chemistry and biology in the late eighteenth and early nineteenth centuries, the way was cleared for a genuine science of pharmacology.

It is amazing that experience-derived complex drug lore was so early codified. The great Ebers Medical Papyrus of about 1550 BC in ancient Egypt seems to have been a teaching formulary. This was a compilation of some nine hundred recommended prescriptions for various diseased conditions indicated by name or brief diagnosis. A modern counterpart is the widely used *Merck Manual* (11th ed., West Point, Pennsylvania, 1966, 1850 pp.). The first compilation of individual drugs considered individually seems to have been made by Dioscorides, the surgeon of Nero, in the first century of our era. This gave names, sources, means of identification, uses and ways of administration with doses. A modern successor is the useful *Merck Index* (8th Ed., Rahway, New Jersey, 1968, 1713 pp.). Today the most widely read reference for information on prescription drugs is the Physician's Desk Reference (PDR). Revised annually, the text material is reviewed by the Food and Drug Administration.

Certain steps were essential for the scientific development of pharmacology and for the rational application of its findings. The first was the need in some way to standardize drug preparations. An initial cooperation between pharmacists and physicians was necessary so that the latter could have some assurance that what they would prescribe would actually be what it was supposed to be. By setting up standards which could be agreed upon, the various drugs could be checked objectively for purity and freedom from adulteration. Physicians could thus begin to have reliance on the probable effects to be produced by a given amount of a drug in an average patient. The Ebers and related early Egyptian medical papyri indicate that this process was under way during the second millenium B.C. The lasting popularity of the compilation of Dioscorides is testimony to its value. The first set of standards for drug preparations to receive legal sanction was the 1546 (Nuremburg) *Dispensatorium* of Valerius Cordus (1515-1544). This was the beginning of modern pharmacopeias.

With quantitative biological techniques, various methods of biological standardization of drugs became possible. These assure uniformity, even now, of various crude drug preparations, such as digitalis, or of various hormones, vaccines, or enzyme products where the chemically pure active ingredient is inconvenient, impossible, or uneconomical to provide. Biological standardization was put on a firm scientific basis by J. H. Burn (1892-1970) when he issued a book with that title (Oxford University Press, 1937, 288 pp.), in application of the classic study on *Statistical Methods for Estimation of Biological Variations in Toxicity Determinations (Proc R Soc [Biol], 101*:483-512, 1927), by the biomathematician, J. W. Trevan (1887-1955).

When A. L. Lavoisier (1743-1794) established quantitative chemical procedures toward the latter part of the eighteenth century, a path opened for the isolation in chemically pure form of the biologically active substances in crude drugs. This was first accomplished by F. W. A. Sertürner (1783-1841) during the early years of the nineteenth century. From the well-known and widely used sleep-producing and pain-relieving drug, opium, he isolated white crystals which caused sleep in his experimental dogs. This substance, of uniform physical and chemical properties, he called *morphine,* from the Graeco-Roman god of sleep, Morpheus. It was the first alkaloid to be extracted from a crude plant source (*J Pharm, 14:47-93,* 1806). This example was promptly followed, under the stimulus of Magendie, by the isolation of many other pure chemical substances from crude biologically active products, and the process continues, as in the case of hormones and immune preparations.

The introduction of pure chemicals as therapeutic agents developed slowly, and yet Magendie soon was able to issue a *Formulaire pour la préparation et l'emploi de plusieurs nouveaux médicaments* (Paris, Mequignon-Marvis, 1822) referring only to elements, inorganic salts and alkaloids. An alert pharmaceutical industry helped. Physicians began to appreciate the physicochemical uniformity and constancy of the pure chemicals made available by such companies as Merck in Germany and Squibb in the United States.

Soon, however, difficulties arose. None of the alkaloids and other compounds recently extracted from crude plant sources were ideal for desired medicinal uses. Often they were too toxic. Chemists tried to characterize these complex compounds in a rational chemical manner. This effort was aided in the case of some organic compounds by the idea of a carbon ring structure as visualized by F. A. Kekule (1829-1896). Yet the attempt was found to be surprisingly difficult. It has been satisfactorily solved only with the past few decades. Thus, morphine was isolated in chemically pure form a century before its chemical constitution was agreed upon. Many chemical relatives close to the natural products were synthesized, however, and some were found to be clinically useful.

Thus, with standardized and uniformly prepared crude drugs on the one hand, and with chemically pure compounds with unvarying physicochemical properties on the other, a way opened for the systematic comparison and evaluation of their biological actions. Thus modern pharmacology could begin. Quickly procedures were developed by physiological and biochemical as well as by pathological techniques, to explore the various biological interactions with drugs: the quantitative toxicity of a drug on a single or repeated administration, with details of symptoms often suggesting the main features of its biological activity; the rate data on its absorption into, its fate within, and its removal from the living material with which it comes in contact; its general biological activity at the various levels of organization of living material from macromolecules to ecologies, and any particular or specific biological effect it may possess. With reference to a similar evaluation of its chemical relatives, rational indication for its various uses may emerge. These then may be tested on human volunteers or under field conditions, and appropriate conclusions may then be drawn for the rational clinical or field use of the drug, as distinct from its empirical use. One may easily diagram this evolutionary development of pharmacology, as I did years ago in an essay entitled "Prolegomenon to Current Pharmacology" (*University of California Publications in Pharmacology, I*:1-29, 1938).

It is clear that the rational use of a drug by the health professions, in agriculture, or in other ways is dependent on the coordinated research endeavors of many kinds of scientists, chiefly chemists, pharmacologists and clinicians. Also possible to be diagramed is the interplay, with feedback effect, of the efforts of these characteristic groups in the development of drugs. These also appropriately are the ones on whom the general public must rely for satisfactory advice on the rational use of a drug and for effective control of its possible abuse.

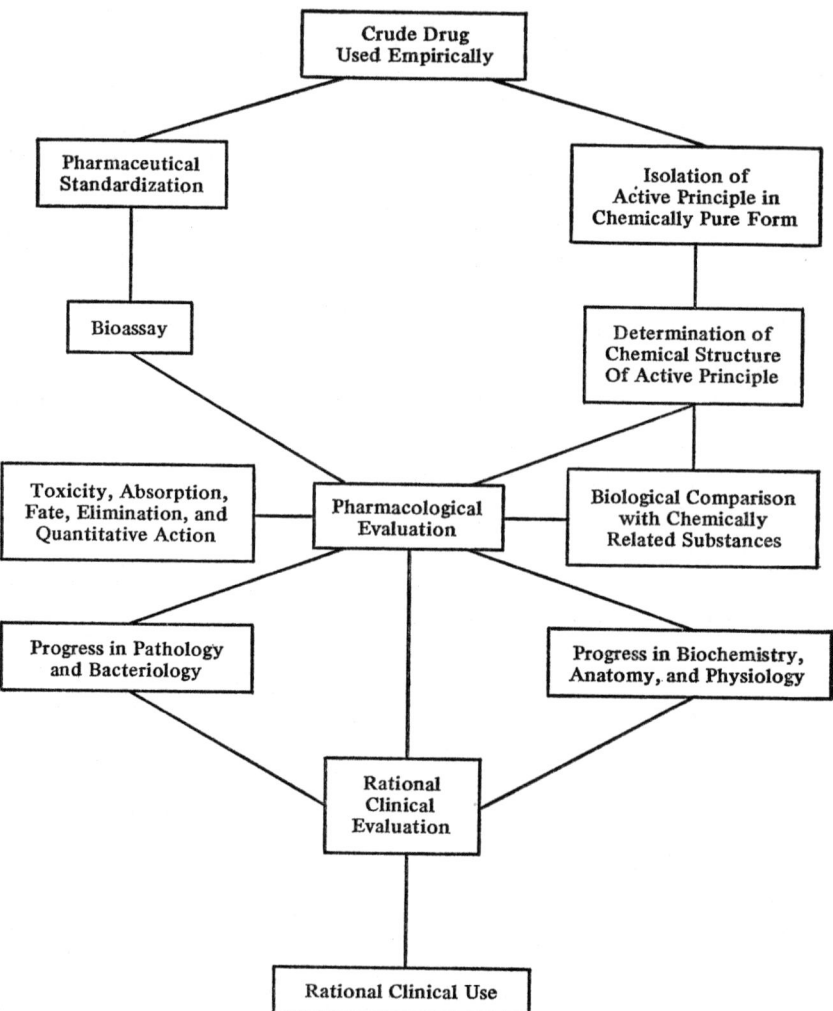

Figure 1-1. The logical and historical position of pharmacology in the rational use of chemical agents in medicine. [Modified from C. D. Leake, "The Pharmacologic Evaluation of New Drugs," *JAMA,* 93:1632-1634 (Nov. 23, 1929)].

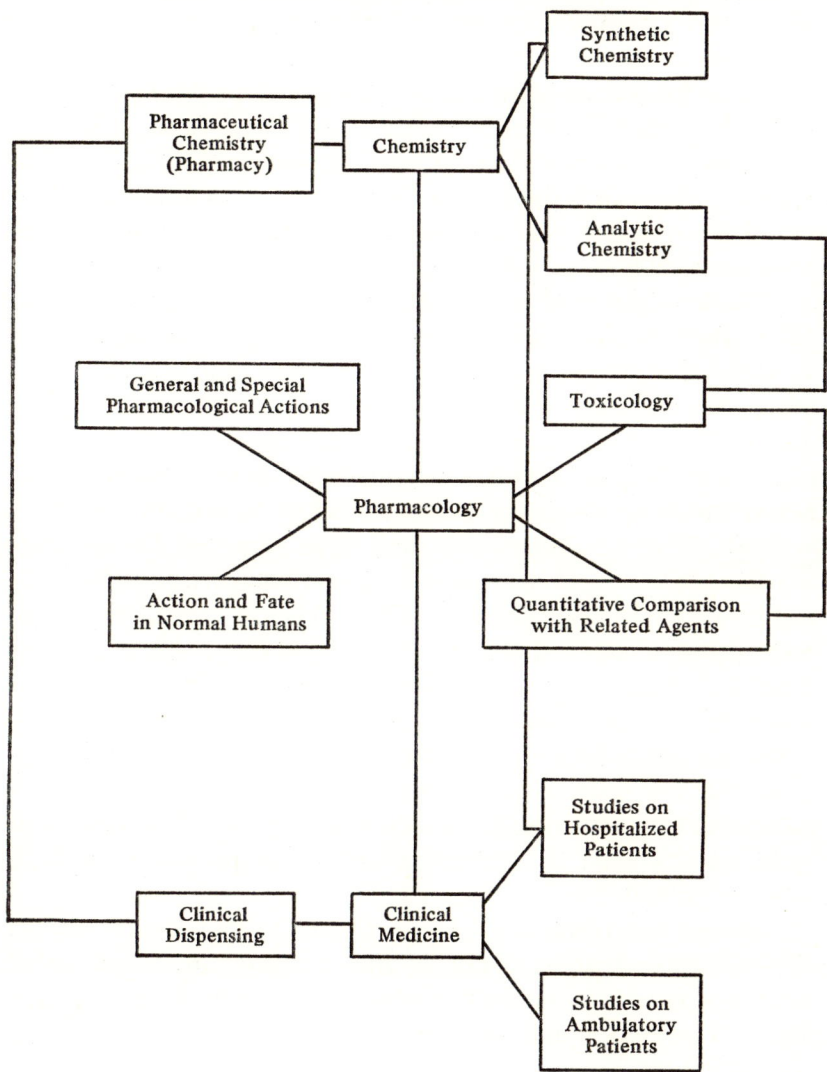

Figure 1-2. Division of labor in the introduction of new chemicals for diagnostic, therapeutic, or prophylactic use in medicine. [From C. D. Leake, "The Pharmacologic Evaluation of New Drugs," *JAMA,* 93:1632-1634 (Nov. 23, 1929)].

Histories of pharmacology have generally been histories of pharmacy. Pharmacology may be considered to be the science; pharmacy is the art. The art of collecting, codifying, and preparing drugs for the use of members of the health professions is much older than any science on the matter could have been. It is interesting that the oldest document relating pharmacy with one of the health professions is the Kahun Egyptian papyrus of around 2,000 BC which contains prescriptions for veterinary medicine along with some for diseases of women.

The first historical account of drugs was made by G. Guibourt (1790-1867) in his *Histoire Abrégée des Drogues Simples* (Paris, L. Colas, 2 volumes, 1820). One of the very best and most complete commentaries on the drugs used in Graeco-Roman, Muslim, and Medieval times is to be found in the translations of the works of Paul of Aegina (625-690 AD) made by Francis Adams (*The Seven Books of Paulus Aegineta,* London Sydenham Society, 3 volumes, 1844-47). About this same time appeared *De Historica Medicamentorum,* (Luchtmans, Lugduni Batavorum, 1846) written by C. P. van der Hoeven (1792-1871). A careful history of local drugs of interest was *Pharmacographia: A History of the Principal Drugs of Vegetable Origin, Met with in Great Britain and British India* (London, Macmillan, 1874), compiled by F. A. Flückiger (1828-1894) and D. Hanbury (1825-1875). There also came the still useful *Bibliotheca Therapeutica . . . Chiefly in Reference to Articles of the Materia Medica* (London, New Sydenham Society, 2 volumes, 1878-79), as prepared by E. J. Waring (1819-1891).

Histories of pharmacy now proliferated. The second edition of *Garrison & Morton's Medical Bibliography,* an indispensable reference source (New York Argosy, 1954), included a thorough listing. The more important are:

Adlung, A., and Urdang, G.: *Grundriss der Geschichte der Deutscher Pharmazie.* Berlin, Springer, 1935.

Andre-Pontier, L.: *Histoire de la Pharmacie.* Paris, Doin, 1900.

Barrett, C.R.B.: *The History of the Society of Apothecaries of London.* London, Elliot Stock, 1905.

Bell, J., and Redwood, T.: *Historical Sketch of the Progress of Pharmacy in Great Britain*. London, Butler & Tanner, 1880.

Benedicenti, A.: *Malati Medici e Farmacisti*. Milano, Hoepli, 2 volumes, 1924-1925.

Berendes, J.: *Geschichte des Pharmacie*. Leipzig, Gunther, 1898.

Boussel, P.: *Histoire Illustree de la Pharmacie*. Paris, Le Prat, 1949.

de Rosemont, L.R.: *Histoire de la Pharmacie à travers les Ages*. Paris, Peyronnet, 1931.

Greer, J.: *A History of Pharmacy*. London, Pharmaceutical Press, 1937.

Kremers, E., and Urdang, G.: *History of Pharmacy*, 3rd ed. Philadelphia, Lippincott, 1963.

LaWall, G.H.: *Four Thousand Years of Pharmacy*. Philadelphia, Lippincott, 1927, (a semi-popular account).

Peters, H.: *Aus Pharmazeutischer Vorzeit in Bild and Wort*. Berlin, Springer, 2 vols., 1889-1891.

Schelenz, H.: *Geschichte der Pharmacie*. Berlin, Springer, 1904 (most comprehensive and informative of all).

Thompson, C.J.S.: *The Mystery and Art of the Apothecary*. London, John Land, 1929.

Wootton, A.C.: *Chronicles of Pharmacy*. London, Macmillan, 2 vols., 1910.

Several accounts and lists of herbals have much historical interest for the history of pharmacology. Notable are the following:

Arber, A.R.: *Herbals: Their Origin and Evolution*. Cambridge, University Press, 1938.

Dragendorff, G.J.N.: *Die Heilpflanzen der verschiedenen Volker und Zeiten*. Stutgart, F. Enke, 1898.

Klebs, A.C.: *Catalogue of Early Herbals*. Lugano, l'art ancien.

Rohde, E.S.: *The Old English Herbals*. London, Longmans, Green, 1922.

Singer, C.J.: *The Herbal in Antiquity and Its Transmission to Later Ages*. In Studies, J.H.: *47*:1-52, 1927. (Dr. Singer was a great historian of science and medicine; his writings are delightful and informative and well-illustrated).

A special report on the development of pharmacopeias was made by George Urdang for the World Health Organization (*Bull WHO, 4*:577-603, 1951). One of the most important but little-known series of historical studies on pharmacology came through the stimulus of Eduard Rudolf Kobert (1854-1918), professor both of the history of medicine and of pharmacology at the University of Dorpat. This is a five-part set of publications, edited by Kobert entitled *Historische Studien aus dem Pharmakologischen Institute der Kaiserlichen Universitat Dorpat* (Tausch & Grosse, Halle). Part I (1889) has 266 pages; Part II (1890) has 181 pages; Part III (1893) has 481 pages; Part IV (1894) has 295 pages, and the final Part V (1896) has 323 pages, for a total of 1546 pages.

The extraordinary scope of Kobert's effort is indicated merely by the titles of some of the articles inspired by him. The first part of the *Studien*, for example, contains his own history of ergot as a drug, used and abused; a discussion of the pharmacological knowledge indicated in the Hippocratic writings, by R. von Grot, and a detailed account of Russian folk-medicine by W. Demetisch. The third part gives the translation and commentary of the materia medica text of Abu Mansur Muwaffak bin Ali Harawi of 1055 AD, by Abdul-Chalig Achundow of Daku, with an important bibliography of historical writings on pharmacology. The fourth part contains further studies on Russian folk-medicine by A. A. Henrici, of Helsingfors, and material on Lettish folk-medicine by J. Alksnis of Kurland. The fifth part contains a translation of the first century BC formulary of Scribonius Largus, with commentary, and then a remarkable description of beer, with details on its making with and without hops and its uses as a vehicle and as a medicinal agent, by the modest editor himself. Kobert must have been a brilliant and inspiring teacher to have obtained so many excellent historical studies from his pupils and colleagues. It is quite unfortunate that these very significant studies seem to have been so generally ignored by medical historians.

Charles C Thomas, Springfield, Illinois, has sponsored a series of well-chosen and well-illustrated classic reports of historical significance in biomedical development. These are: *Selected Readings in Pathology*, issued in 1929 by Esmond R. Long; *Selected Readings in the History of Physiology* first published in 1930, with John F. Fulton (1899-1963) as author, and *Classic Descriptions of Disease* by Ralph H. Major, first offered in 1932, and in testimony of its excellence, many times reprinted in several editions. To these now have been added *Readings in Pharmacology,* selected and edited by B. Holmstedt and G. Liljestrand of Stockholm (Oxford, Pergamon Press, 1963). The biographical sketches and illustrations in this volume are particularly helpful. Yet there seems to me to be many unfortunate omissions. Selection, however, is a personally biased activity.

A smaller selection of mostly current classic contributions to pharmacology, with slight technical commentary, was made by Louis Shuster of Boston *(Readings in Pharmacology,* Boston, Little, Brown & Co., 1962). A rather extensive symposium covering an *Ethnopharmacologic Search for Psychoactive Drugs* was edited by D. H. Efron (National Institute for Mental Health, Public Health Service Publication 1645, Washington, D.C., 1967). R. N. Chopra gave a full account of *Indigenous Drugs of India: Their Medical and Economic Aspects* (Calcutta, The Art Press, 1933).

The story of pharmacological development is so interesting and actually exciting that it is certain to have a popular appeal. Several popular accounts of pharmacology are available. One of the best is *Magic in a Bottle* (New York, Macmillan, 1941), by my good friend and colleague, the keen science writer, Milton Silverman. This skillfully relates the intellectual triumphs in the rise of pharmacology during the past two centuries. It is accurate in detail as the careful bibliography attests.

Another example of excellent reporting of the broad background of pharmacology is *Green Medicine: The Search for Plants that Heal* (Chicago, Rand McNally, 1964; New York, Bantam Books, 1966), by another brilliant science writer, Margaret Kreig. This recounts her own dramatic effort to trace the development of pharmacological knowledge from the native use of crude drugs to the sophisticated exploitation of synthetic chemicals derived from their active ingredients.

An example of the slick journalistic approach, with enlarged and arty illustrations, is the Life Science Library item, *Drugs* (New York, Time, 1967), by the vigorous New York pharmacologist Walter Modell, abetted by the freelance writer Alfred Lansing, and the anonymous but strongly patterned ex-editors of

Life. This gives the conventional picture of pharmacology as viewed in the United States.

To all of these sources relating to the history of pharmacology I am deeply indebted. I have myself been witness to much of the recent rapid growth of pharmacological knowledge, and I am personally very grateful to many pharmacological friends in all parts of the world for information and advice on historical matters relating to the science. Mostly my point of view is not a conventional choice of what is significant in the history of pharmacology. Thus, I think that the influence of the German precisionists toward the latter part of the nineteenth century has been greatly overrated in comparison with the generally neglected accomplishments of the Parisian determinists of fifty years earlier.

Pharmacology is a fascinating subject. Firmly grounded now in the fundamental scientific disciplines of mathematics, physics, and chemistry, it has been allied with all the great emerging biomedical sciences, and its applications are extending widely in many ways. Its history cannot fail but be interesting and also significant.

CHAPTER 2

PROTOPHARMACOLOGY: PREHISTORIC EMPIRICAL DRUG LORE

> The Lord hath created medicines out of the earth; and he that is wise will not abhor them.
>
> *Ecclesiasticus* 38:4

A DISCUSSION OF THE HISTORY of pharmacology can easily be divided into two parts: protopharmacology, mostly empirical, but developed by painstaking observation, cultural recording, analysis, and rational application, and pharmacology as a scientific discipline which could only arise with the development of modern chemistry and biology in the nineteenth century of our era.

There has ever been an aura of mystery about drug action and use. It is not surprising then that there are many instances of magical irrationality in the progress of protopharmacology, and that such wishful thinking occurs even now in relation to the achievements of modern pharmacology. Actually, however, there are no miracle drugs. Chemical agents can merely make living material do more or less what it is already capable of doing. There is the danger that either too much or too little may be toxic.

People everywhere on earth have tried the plant, animal and mineral materials in their environment for possible use as food or they have perhaps examined such things from mere curiosity. These things, from fruits, leaves, barks and roots, to fresh or well-hung flesh, blood, viscera, and skins, and earth or minerals of various kinds, have been tasted, smelled, felt, rubbed on the skin, and applied to various orifices of the body. Their effects or sensations were noted and talked about. Ideas about these things were gradually passed along in families. Thus arose the basis for an oral tribal tradition. Gradually such materials that were especially liked, e.g. foods, or as might cause desired effects such as purging, were recognized. Unusual effects on ingestion or skin application were slowly applied, often quite logically, to produce such effects as might be thought useful in treating illness and in promoting health. Thus some of these naturally occurring materials became used as drugs, i.e. agents for the management of disease and injury.

In this way, tribal folklore on drugs probably slowly accumulated. Intertribal communication may have gradually promoted exchange of such drug products as were to be found in special local communities. Thus, common salt was an article of early extensive trade between inland forest areas, as in Europe and North America, and hot dry places near the sea where salt deposits were found. The salt trade-routes were well established on the major continents long before any recorded history. It is remarkable that salt was so generally and so early appreciated as being essential for good health. Perhaps the observation of the use of salt-licks by animals may have been a factor in this recognition. Likewise fresh water was sought from springs, desert water-holes, and snow-water in the polar regions, not only for slaking thirst but also for cooling and refreshing the skin. Springs were revered as sacred places coming from the good earth which gave nourishment and life.

Observations on what animals eat in their environment may have influenced the human choice of foods. It is interesting to reflect that diet still remains an important factor in preventing disease and in promoting good health. Various foods seem to have been scrutinized for their possible health value early, and those who slowly rose to be the health advisors, wise ones or priests, were expected to know the health qualities of foods and to advise about their use. The extant records of early health leaders in China, India, Sumeria, Egypt, and ancient Greece are full of dietary suggestions, often with much detail regarding the presumed benefits to be obtained from every known variety of fruit, grain, berry, vegetable or tuber.

When the eating of certain plants was noted to be followed

by purgation, these plants, or the parts of them thought to be most active, gradually came to be used deliberately to induce purgation when individuals were constipated. Sometimes these kinds of plants were used for ritualistic purging at periodic tribal rites, and thus may be said to have been used for social purposes. Similarly, other plants or parts of them whose ingestion might be followed by vomiting were often directly employed to induce emesis in order to get rid of unpleasant feeling of an overloaded stomach, and again, in some tribal rites for ritualistic vomiting.

Thus, aloes, asafetida, bryonia, butternut, cassia, colocynth, elaterium, figs, frangula, manna, olive oil, podophyllum, prunes, senna, sulfur, and tamarind, as well as other plant materials became widely used as purges under early prehistoric conditions among the various tribes clustering around the Mediterranean basin and other centers of growing culture.

Even as late as the mid-nineteenth century of our era, the natives in the Cascade mountains of northwestern North America were found to have learned of the purgative properties of the bark of an indigenous tree, cascara sagrada *(Rhamnus purshiana)*. It was only then that this safe and effective laxative was incorporated into current medical practice. It is interesting that a preparation of the crude bark, fluid-extract of cascara, is preferable to the chemically pure active principle, the anthroquinone glucoside, emodin. The latter is too irritating to the bowel, but the gums, resins, and tannins in the crude preparation reduce the local irritation of the active principle, delay its effectiveness, and thus make it more gentle and satisfactory.

People everywhere found barks of trees which would help them to control diarrhea. Barks, as we know now, contain the astringent, mild antiseptic, tannin, which is effective in reducing bacterial irritation of bowels. Many such barks were later thought to be highly specific for amebic dysentery, but their usefulness is merely due to the nonspecific tannin which they contain. Constipation and diarrhea or dysentery are the two antithetical conditions afflicting most people at some time or other. It is significant that indigenous people everywhere on earth learned very early of the plant purgatives and of the bark antidiarrheals in their neighborhoods. These materials had been tried for food, and their effects had been noted; probably after much trial and debate these effects were rationally applied to practical conditions.

Larch agaric and chamomile were used anciently as emetics in the proto-european cultures. The vomiting nut, *nux vomica*, of India, Indo-China and Australia, had long been used for emesis in these areas before coming into European medical practice. Ipecac root was found by the Brazilian Itenez River natives to cause vomiting and was ritualistically used by them for this purpose long before it was introduced into European medicine in the seventeenth century.

Pain must have been as much a mystery and agony to early people as it is to us. Many ways were found to relieve pain. I once tried to tell the story in *Letheon: The Cadenced Story of Anesthesia* (Austin, University of Texas Press, 1947):

> In every place the people tasted this or that
> in seeking what they might with safety eat,
> and learned what each might do
> to bowel or head or heart.
> What cooled the fiery, painful skin they noted, too,
> and learning, treasured deep and long in memory.
> So when desire rose to alter bowel
> to dull the ache of head or heart,
> or soothe the flushed and irritated skin,
> remembrance showed the way.
> What Bachic genius first found joy in fruit juice
> as worked upon by warming sun?
> Each tribe preserved the mythic hints
> of earthy Dionysan secrets, which
> suggested peace from frenzied want.
> Peace came with wines and human sympathy.
>
> The soothing voice and touch came first,
> then food, and oily balm,
> then skill, as taught by Imhotep,
> to set the broken bone,
> to calm the fiery skin, –
> the quiet hand of Susruta,
> the cooling lotions of Egyptian priests,
> the wine Hua-Tu devised to stupify with hemp,
> the skillful pressure on the nerves

and vessels to a limb,
or on the ones still called "carotids,"
the arteries of sleep which pulse in neck, –
the Scythian hemp, the Memphic stone,
the *sama* of Hebraic surgeon-priests,
the Persian wines,
the temple-sleep in ancient Greece,
the vinegars of crucified, –
these were all known somewhere
to dull the hurt of injury.
And some were used to blunt the senses,
when the healing priest performed his rite,
or cut away the cancer or the rotted part
with stone or bronze scalpel.

The wines and beers themselves were early found
to be of comfort in an agony,
and to them many herbs
were added by the priestly surgeons everywhere:
The lotus, lettuce, mandrake, poppy, dock,
the henbane, hemlock, hellebore and hemp,
verbana, primrose, myrrh and frankincense,
the deadly nightshade, garlic, bhang,
and half around the world
where other people learned, –
the kava, mescal, leaves of coca and tobacco, –
these and many more
kept secret, unidentified,
comprise the ancient anodynes.

Many useful drugs came into conventional medical practice during the seventeenth century, from various places in Latin America and Africa, where the natives had long before discovered their potential medical value. Among such drugs were coca leaves and Peruvian bark from the Andes, from which were isolated in the nineteenth century such active substances as cocaine and quinine respectively. From Africa came the ordeal bean, *Physostigma venenosum*, from which the alkaloid physostigmine was isolated by Jobst and Hesse in 1864. From Africa also came the seeds of a vine, *Strophanthus*, used to calm the heart, and finally from this the glucoside strophanthin was isolated in the nineteenth century. From nux vomica was obtained the alkaloid strychnine and from ipecac came the alkaloid emetine.

Prehistoric drug lore reveals many examples of wisdom in applying observable phenomena to desired ends. Thus, the upper Amazonian natives discovered that a gummy stuff from the bark of a certain tree would paralyze an animal if stuck through its skin, but that it was harmless if taken by mouth. This gummy stuff was called curare, wooari, or urari, words which according to Margaret Kreig's exciting account in *Green Medicine* means "he, to whom it comes, falls." This was widely used as an arrow poison. It was shown in an experimental study (*Bull Gen Ther, 69*:23-25, 1865) by famed Claude Bernard (1813-1878) that it blocks nerve transmission at the neuromuscular junction.

When the plant source was finally identified by B. A. Krukoff of the New York Botanical Garden as *Chondodendron tomentosum,* a woody vine, the way was cleared for scientific extraction from it of the alkaloid, d-tubocurarine by O. Winterstein in 1943 at the Squibb Research Laboratories. A clinical study by A. R. McIntyre of the University of Nebraska (*Curare,* Chicago, University of Chicago Press, 1947, 240 pp.) revealed its usefulness in various spastic disorders and its ability to cause muscular relaxation in anesthesia.

Biochemorphic considerations led to important synthetic derivatives. It had been shown by A. C. Brown (1839-1923) and T. R. Fraser (1841-1920) that various alkaloids with tertiary nitrogen and differing biological activities uniformly acquire a curare-like action through conversion to quaternary ammonium bases. Reasoning on this relationship resulted in the development of decamethonium compounds for muscular relaxation. Calabash curare is obtained from the *Strychnos toxifera* vine; many muscle relaxing alkaloids have been isolated from this by Paul Karrer (1889-1972) in Zürich. One, toxiferine, is widely used in Europe to relax muscles.

The ancient Greeks used willow barks and leaves crushed in olive oil to apply to rheumatic or arthritic joints or muscles. Arthritis was common in antiquity in the Near East as old Egyptian mummy bones testify. Willow (Salix) contains a glucoside called salicin; its chemical make-up led to the synthesis of salicylic acid. Its many derivatives, chief of which is aspirin (acetyl-salicylic acid), are used the world over for the relief of rheumatic and arthritic aches and pains. The Amerinds of the eastern United States used crushed leaves of wintergreen for the same purpose. We now know that oil of wintergreen is methyl salicylate and is often used in ointments to help reduce the pain of rheumatism and arthritis.

It must have been anciently noted in many parts of the world that mashed fruits, berries or grain allowed to lie in warm sunlight would soon acquire peculiar tastes and would produce effects when ingested which would be quite different from the original. The making of beers was already a skilled technical procedure in ancient Egypt as early as 3,000 BC as indicated by later clay-figurines of the beermakers and carbon dating of relics of some of the equipment used. The high level of technique achieved is suggested by the indicated methods of clarification. Beer was often used as a vehicle for medicaments and was recognized as having diuretic properties in itself.

Grapes do not grow readily in too hot a climate, but wines seem also to have been made at very early times in the northeast Mediterranean basin. In his pleasant account of *A History of Wine as Therapy* (Philadelphia, Lippincott, 1963, 234 pp.), Salvatore P. Lucia quotes extensively from Homer and the Old Testament to indicate the antiquity of the use of wines. Their power to relieve suppurating wounds was recognized, and they were widely employed in surgical dressings. They were known to cause relaxation and a tendency to sleep. They also stimulated the appetite. Often resins were used to prevent wines from spoiling, and such resinated wines survive now in Greece.

Wines were thought to contain a spirit which could inspire, or with too much, intoxicate. As J. G. Frazer suggested in *The Golden Bough* (New York, Macmillan, 5 volumes, 1935), wines were also considered to be the blood of the grape, and thus to contain the spirit of the grape. As Lucia shows, wines were used medicinally as well as for beverage purposes in ancient India and China. The Old Testament account of the drunkenness of Noah is an ancient legend indicating that there was an early appreciation of possible abuses of wine drinking.

The tranquilizing and relaxing properties of beers and wines seem to have been recognized as relieving tensions and promoting social unity. They could thus have been important factors in advancing intertribal communication and thus in helping to develop civilization. There was also early recognition that excessive intake would cause incoherent and unsatisfactory behavior. Thus, there seems to have been an appreciation of a simple fact about drugs; a little bit may be beneficial; a little bit more may be harmful. Wines were used ritualistically in social ceremonies among most ancient peoples. Thus, there was some degree of social control over their possible abuse.

Such social control over drug use was especially significant in early tribal societies in regard to hallucinating agents. These were found in all parts of the world by local natives seeking food in their environments. From Siberia to Mexico certain mushrooms were discovered to be amazingly effective in causing scintillating visions of euphoric bliss.

The resin and leaves of the widely dispersed hemp were used in many parts of the world to produce relaxed dreaming. In the South Pacific the pithy kava root was chewed for its mild relaxing effects. Among the Amerinds, tobacco leaves and other mild euphoriates, as lobelia, were smoked to give a feeling of restful peace.

Importantly, wherever agents of this sort were found, their use was generally ritualized by the priestly tribal leaders so that the social community together would partake of the pleasure or inspiration induced by these various euphoric drugs. Thus, the possibility of individual abuse was greatly reduced. At the same time, the common exulting experience produced a sense of social or communal unity.

In antiquity an individual abuser of hallucinating drugs was ridiculed as the legend of Noah suggests. A tribal group would never have tolerated drug abuse.

Gordon Wasson has given the most succinct statement of the wide use of the fly agaric mushroom, *Amanita muscaria* (in *Ethnopharmacologic Search for Psychoactive Drugs*. Washington, D.C., US Natl. Inst. Mental Health, 1967. pp. 405-451). He describes its long use among various Siberian tribes, including the serial drinking of the urine of previous eaters in order to get the euphoric effect second hand, an unusual observation of urinary excretion of a potent drug. The antiquity of the use of this hallucinating mushroom is indicated by probable reference to it in old Sanskirt vedas.

Robert Graves, the great nonconforming poet, has also speculated much on the ancient use of hallucinating mushrooms. He thinks the tremendous physical feats of the primitive Greek moon-worshiping maenads, and even of the Biblical hero, Samson, were induced by wines laced with mushrooms. Even the Vikings were supposed to have gone "berserk" in this manner. The extreme physical relaxation coming after the initial excitement caused by the drug could result in defeat, as the legend of Samson suggests. The Vikings stopped the *berserkvorgang* in the tenth century. Margaret Kreig gives a good account of the anthropological studies of the Wassons on hallucinating mushrooms in Mexico (*Green Medicine,* New York, Bantam Books, 1966, pp. 261-268).

Margaret Kreig offers many interesting and exciting accounts of the indigenous development of crude drugs serving many useful purposes, as found in the environments of ancient people, often mistakenly called *primitive*. Many of these ancient drugs are currently significant and will be discussed as their scientific development fits into modern chronology. Among such drugs are cinchona bark, digitalis, chaulmoogra, sarsaparilla, yams, snakeroot, periwinkles, oloiuqui, and even drugs from the sea.

Kava, *Piper methysticum,* about which Louis Lewin (1850-1929) wrote so well in his famed *Phantastica* (Berlin G. Stilke, 1924) is well discussed in *Ethnopharmacologic Search for Psychoactive Drugs,* edited by D. H. Efron (Washington, D.C., Nat. Inst. Mental Health, 1967, pp. 105-181). Nutmeg *(Myristica fragrans)* and various South American snuffs are also fully considered in this same volume. Francisco Guerra, the Spanish pharmacologist and medical historian, has collected information on some twenty hallucinating Mexican crude drugs in his *Las Plantas Fantasticas de Mexico* (Mexico City, Diario Espanol, 1954, 122 pp.). Their use is pre-Colombian in origin.

As Margaret Kreig emphasizes, the empirical development of useful crude drugs in the environments of primitive people was usually accompanied and often superseded by magical rituals. These reflected the wishful effort to achieve what was desired from the unknown surrounding powers of good and evil, either by shamanistically propitiating angry forces, driving out or frightening away evil influences, or cajoling indifferent fateful powers for benefit, individually in sickness, or tribally in epidemics. In the absence of any clear knowledge of the causes of infections or metabolic diseases, this recourse to magic was reasonable.

It is amazing to note how persistent some of these anciently used crude drugs and health-giving foods are, knowledge of the presumed virtues of which are still treasured in folklore. Even in our sophisticated society, there is still a growing cult of natural food faddists, especially among our youth. These natural foods are supposed to contribute to good health. In many cases they are carry-overs from antiquity. Those who grow their own vegetables and fruits in order to avoid pesticides, artificial fertilizers, or growth-promoting contaminants often follow the ancient ritual of planting during a waxing moon and harvesting as the moon wanes. Natural food stores are thriving in our large cities.

Wisely it would seem that from antiquity people have been as interested in preserving good health as in relieving the symptoms of disease. People everywhere seem to realize that proper and adequate food, with as much variety as possible, is necessary for health. In every part of the world, native dietaries developed from the indigenous plants in the area which supplied essential nutriments. Both food and drugs were realized as being involved in health.

Many crude drugs seem to have been promoted in antiquity on the basis of imagined similarities to what was desired. This doctrine of signatures would suggest, for instance, that in obvious blood lack, in a pale anemic person, the ingestion of red rusty iron particles would be helpful; the red of the rust going with the red of the blood. Red wine would be thought to be useful for the same reason. This would occur, in the case of iron, long before there was any demonstrable reason in a modern scientific sense to believe that blood contains iron. Yet, the belief was there.

Similarly, the roots of ginseng or mandragora, the mandrakes of Biblical lore, were thought to resemble the human body with their bulbous shape and paired appendages. Such beliefs about ginseng persist now in China and once furnished a lucrative income to Wisconsin farmers who exported quantities of the roots to satisfy Chinese demands. Russian scientists now claim to have found blood-pressure altering agents in ginseng.

As Douglas Guthrie has said (*Trans Bot Soc Edin, 39*:184-195, 1961) of the "doctrine of signatures": "For every disease, it was argued, God had provided a remedy, and the only problem was how to find it." The clue lay in the plant itself. Saffron, with its yellow color, was the cure for jaundice. *Pulmonaria,* which had marking on its leaves resembling the lungs, would cure lung disease. Cyclamen had a leaf like the human ear: "it was the remedy for ear disorders."

The accumulation and development of local drug lore was part of the general culturalization process of the community. This was related to and included in the gradual domestication of plants for food use, the slow taming of beasts to form flocks and herds, and the highly complicated ways of handling metals. Each was probably a family oriented procedure with techniques handed down through generations. It was associated with the growth of skills in weaving, pottery making, and other basic home arts. Those who become proficient in gathering herbs for the preparation of drugs for use in caring for the sick become the early druggists. Drug lore was an essential part of the process of civilization.

Myths from all areas provide much information about the folklore of drugs. The most comprehensive study of myths is the great compilation of James George Frazer (1854-1941) in his *The Golden Bough* (London, 12 volumes, 1911-1915). The Greek myths have been well analyzed, documented, and annotated by the English poet, Robert Graves, (*The Greek Myths,* Baltimore, Penguin Books, 1955, 2 volumes).

Graves refers to aconite, the tuberous roots of monkshood,

wolf's bane, or mouse-bane, *Aconitum napellus,* of the Ranunculaceae, found in the mountains of Europe and Asia. This contains about 1 percent of several active substances, including the powerfully poisonous alkaloid, aconite. Graves says, "Aconite, a poison and paralysant, was used by Thessalonian witches in making their flying ointment,"—it numbs feet and hands to give a sensation of being off the ground. But since it is a febrifuge, Heracles, who drove away the fever-birds from Stymphalus, was credited with its discovery." Aconite continued to be used for centuries to treat fevers and strengthen hearts. It continued in use to induce the "Witches Sabbath." as described by Merejkowski in his description of the Walpurgis Night in his *Romance of Leonardo.*

Some idea of the drugs and spices used in the bronze age Minoan and Mycenean cultures is emerging from the deciphering of the "Linear B" clay inventory tablets from Knossus by M. Ventris and J. Chadwick (*Documents in Mycenean Greek,* University of Cambridge Press, 1956). As given by C. P. W. Warren (*Med Hist, 14*:364-377, 1970), these are similar to the various drugs and condiments recommended in the several old Egyptian medical papyri. Since Knossus was probably destroyed by the volcanic explosion of Santorini around 1400 BC, it seems likely that there was borrowing from the earlier Egyptian codified folklore medicine. Yet, the supposed virtues of these same plant remedies may have been independently discovered by the Cretans, and then passed onto the Greek tradition to be mentioned in the Homeric poems and later by Theophrastus, and finally to be embalmed for medieval use in the compilation of Dioscorides in the first century AD.

As listed by Warren, the plants with medicinal properties noted in the Knossus tablets were celery, coriander, cumin, Cyperus grass, dates, fennel, figs, garden cress, ginger, iris root, linseed, mint, pennyroyal, rose, safflower (seed?), sage and sesame (seed?). Found in archeological sites are onion, garlic, poppy-seed and saffron. Most of these we would consider to be condiments. Yet in the bronze age they may have been used as much for their presumed health-giving powers as for flavoring of foods.

No indication is given in the Knossus tablets of medicinal use. Some of the plants inventoried such as figs and linseed, are mildly cathartic. Iris root may have been used for cardiotonic effect. Garlic and onion are mildly antiseptic and are soothing for insect bites. It is not to be thought that the finding of the poppy seed is indicative of the use of opium. This powerful soporific and pain-relieving agent was not known until about our era. It is strange that hemp is not listed since its depressant action was known at that time. Certainly wine and beer were also known but seem not to have been included in the inventories.

Much of scientific value and perhaps even of clinical interest remains hidden in the vast folklore about drugs. The large dispensatory volumes, still popular at the beginning of our century, contain much information of this sort. Still useful is such a huge compilation as that made by H. A. Hare (1862-1931), Charles Caspari Jr. (1850-1917) and H. H. Rusby (1855-1940) in *The National Standard Dispensatory* (Philadelphia, Lea & Febiger, 3rd ed., 1916, 2081 pp.). There still is need for a systematic exploration of folklore medicine in order to derive from it what might yet be useful for us.

CHAPTER 3

PROTOPHARMACOLOGY: CODIFIED EMPIRICAL DRUG USE

> A drug is a substance that, when injected into a rat, produces a scientific paper.
>
> EDGERTON Y. DAVIS, JR.

MOST OF THE GREAT STATIC cultures of antiquity were already well established when records began to be kept. Some kind of agreed-upon system of symbols had to be developed for communication. Perhaps initial pictographs became conventionalized, and when given phonetic equivalents, they could become the basis of language, both spoken and written. Records began to be kept of the gradual accumulation of knowledge as early as the fourth millenia BC, in such widely separated areas as China, India, Sumeria and Egypt. Possibly similar developments occurred in Mykenian and Minoan cultures in the pre-Greek era, but the records persist only in myths. It is interesting that a similar culture expression should have occurred much later in Mexico. In all these cases there was codification of drug lore which had been slowly gathered for centuries earlier.

This codification implied an attempt at systematic ordering of material. Some effort had to be made at classification. Our knowledge of the records is incomplete, and indeed, many of the possible records seem to be lost. The resulting material now available ranges from separate drug prescriptions, as in the Sumerian clay tablets, to drug compilations, as found in China and even in Aztec codices, to extensive formularies for the guidance of physicians, as found in the old Egyptian medical papyri.

I will begin my discussion of codified drug lore accumulated through antiquity with a consideration of ancient Chinese codification, then proceed to Hindu classics, then to the Mesopotamian drug records, and the Egyptian medical papyri. This discussion will conclude with comments on Mayan and Aztec compilations. Thus I follow a rough chronological order.

Chinese Drug Lore

China is an immense area and certainly has been populated by highly intelligent people for many millenia. The technical achievements of the Chinese have been particularly well studied by Joseph Needham, the distinguished biochemist of Cambridge University. Since 1954, he has issued seven volumes on *Science and Civilization in China*. Most of this is concerned with the technical achievements of the Chinese, but there is clear evidence of their intellectual skill in organizing the observations which they made.

In her account of the *Yellow Emperor's Classic of Internal Medicine* (Berkeley, University of California Press, 1966, 260 pp.), Ilza Veith refers to Shen-nung as the second of the legendary emperors. He is said to have lived in about what corresponds to 2700 BC. He was called the Divine Husbandman and was venerated as the father of agriculture. As such he is reputed to have tasted all herbs in order to acquaint himself with their possible usefulness. To him is commonly attributed the writing of the great Chinese herbal, the *Pen Tsao*. However, in the dogmatic and ambiguous *Chinese Medicine* by P. Huard and Ming Wong (New York, McGraw-Hill, 1969, 253 pp.), the question is raised as to whether or not Pen Tsao is a person. Yet the symbols *Pen Tsao* are commonly ascribed to the compilation of medicinal herbs that were used from antiquity in China.

The *Pen Tsao* is a classification of medical plants and a codification of mixtures of them for various medicinal purposes. The *Nei-Ching* or the great text of Chinese medicine is ascribed to the Emperor Hant-Ti who lived in what corresponded to about 2700 BC. According to Fielding Garrison, the literary source of Chinese medicine perhaps developed not earlier than the Han

Dynasty. He says that "the making of medicinal decoctions is attributed to I-Yin, a famous prime minister of the Shang Dynasty (1176-1123 BC) ." Garrison goes on to say:

> The *Pen Tsao* and the *Nei-Ching* were done in lacquer upon strips of bamboo or palm leaves. The tadpole characters, derived from the ancient device of making knots in strings, were arranged vertically to accommodate themselves to the narrow bamboo surface. These tadpole ideograms, the analog of the Egyptian picture writings, were later modified and done with pen and paper. The ideogram for 'physician' (pronounced *i*) contains, like the Egyptian hieroglyph, an arrow or a lancet in the upper half and a drug — or bleeding glass — in the lower. In the Han Dynasty, about the beginning of our era, medicine advanced rapidly through recording of clinical cases and the work of Chang Chung-Ching, an author of treatises on dietetics and fevers, and Hua To, the famous surgeon of China, who probably used *Cannabis indica* for anesthesia.

Buddhism was introduced into China about the beginning of our era and led to considerable confusion with Taoism. There was much popular interest in long life and the search for drugs which might prolong life. Much compilation of medical lore continued until the sixteenth century of our era. At that time Li Shi Chen issued a synopsis of ancient herbals that remained popular for a long time.

The maintenance of harmony in health or its restoration in disease provided a theoretical background for Chinese medicine. This postulated the importance in an individual of a balance between the female principle, or ying, and the male principle, or yang. In practice there developed a fantastic number lore with rather exact anthropometry, and an amazing hierarchy of interrelations between the organs and viscera, and the drugs appropriate to each. The Chinese used massage widely and skillfully and introduced the moxa. This consisted of small combustible cones applied to various parts of the body and ignited for relief of fever or local pains. There was wide use of acupuncture. This is the sticking of needles with careful precision into certain parts of the body for counter-irritant action in rheumatic and arthritic pains. Ivory manikins were made to show the exact point of puncture. The Chinese made much of pulse lore, with special drugs to be used in relation to each variation.

The Chinese materia medica is extensive. It includes such well known plant drugs as aloes, aconite, ephedra, ginseng, hemp, pomegranate, rhubarb, senna, and worm-wood, as well as mineral preparations containing arsenic, mercury and sulfur, and parts of animals and excreta. Opium may have been introduced into China from the Mideast sometime about the beginning of our era.

The drug trade in China has always been enormous. Pharmacies thrive and there is much mysticism and secrecy associated with the preparation of prescriptions. Pharmacists dispense directly in accordance with their judgment, and physicians are consulted only in emergencies. Even now, in the Chinatowns of great Western cities one may find the Chinese pharmacies extremely busy. A great many crude plant, animal and mineral materials are neatly arranged for prompt mixture and dispensing in accordance with the opinion of the pharmacist. There seems to be much reliance on the "doctrine of signatures," and on astrological signs and portents. The notion that the horn of the rhinoceros is powerful and thus a potent aphrodisiac is enough to result in the near extinction of the animals by hunters.

From the ancient accumulation of knowledge regarding the medicinal properties of native material in China, some useful modern developments have come. My colleague, Ko-Kui Chen, worked under Harold Bradley in biochemistry and under Arthur Loevenhart in pharmacology at the University of Wisconsin and received his medical degree from Johns Hopkins. He then went to China to teach at Peking Union Medical College, and his avowed purpose in his careful training was to explore the Chinese materia medica, and especially the many herbs noted in the *Pen Tsao* to determine whether or not any of them might be worthy of intensive study by modern pharmacological methods.

Chen noted that a plant called Ma Huang occurred frequently in prescriptions recommended for the treatment of asthma. Upon investigating, he found that Ma Huang is the Chinese name for a desert plant which we identify as *Ephedra vulgaris*. From this plant the alkaloid ephedrine has been isolated. Chen found that the chemical constitution of ephedrine is closely related to that of epinephrine, the chemically active principle from the adrenal medulla which causes vasoconstriction, bronchorelaxation, dilated pupils, and increase in blood sugar, and indeed all the physiological reactions which Walter Cannon (1871-1945) included in the emergency response to sudden stress in preparing an animal for "fight or flight."

Chen realized the ephedrine could be administered by mouth and might be a useful agent for the treatment of asthmatic conditions. He introduced it with C. F. Schmidt as the sulfate for the treatment of asthma. It became widely popular. It was realized further that the drug might have central nervous system stimulating properties. Its subsequent scarcity and high price was what led Gordon Alles (1901-1963), working in our San Francisco laboratory, to try to find a synthetic substitute for it. This effort resulted in the amphetamines.

Chen also found that toad skins were widely used in the Chinese materia medica for cardiac conditions. He was able to isolate several carditonic bufotoxins for cardiac use from such material. He also found that the toad skins contain bufotenin, which has hallucinating properties. Many other workers, among them Bernard Read, have studied the traditional Chinese materia medica and have attempted to find other products that might be clinically useful.

Ginseng is widely used in China for a variety of conditions. It is the root of a plant which has a bulbous center with a little knob at the top, a couple of roots that go out at right angles, and a forked appendage at the bottom. It has something of a human shape. The closer the form comes to that of the human body, the more efficacious the drug is thought to be. It is recommended for long life, as a remedy for arthritis, as an aphrodisiac, and as a general tonic and cure for cancer. It is widely cultivated in the Wisconsin woods and shipped to China. Nothing significantly active has been found in it by conventional pharmacologists. Yet, the Russians recently have claimed that there is a vasoconstricting action in ginseng and that it may relieve depression. Ginseng is one of the most characteristic of Chinese drugs.

Hindu Drugs

The oldest Sanskrit documents dealing with medicine consist of versified spells and incantations against demons of disease. It was not until the millenia preceding ours that a sort of rational medicine developed in India. The Brahman priests and scholars were the major medical leaders. There are three Brahmanical medical texts of importance: (1) *Charaka Samahita,* a compendium made in the second century of our era, but copied from a much earlier work; (2) the *Susrata,* of the fifth century of our era, and (3) the *Vagbahata,* from the seventh century of our era. The *Samahita* was translated by William D. Whitney, and revised by C. R. Lanman (Cambridge, Harvard Oriental Series, Vol. 7-8, 1905). The *Susrata* was translated into English by K. K. Lal (Calcutta, Bhishagratna, 3 volumes, 1907-1916).

While the outstanding feature of Hindu medicine was surgical skill, there was significant achievement in the management of disease even though there was no recognition of a distinction between infectious or metabolic involvement. Various types of illnesses were carefully described. There was a basic theory of disease. It was thought to be a derangement of the proper proportions of the seven fundamental principles of chyle, blood, flesh, fat, bone, marrow, and semen. Little attention was paid to urine. Drugs were proposed for modification or substitution of these principles.

The Hindus were skilled enough to attribute malaria fever to the presence of mosquitos and to associate rats with plague. They recognized diabetes mellitus and they detailed a careful regimen in therapeutics which included baths, enemas, emetics, inhalations, gargles, and many plant drugs by mouth.

There are over seven hundred medicinal plants described by Susrata, some of which were imported from other places. There was widespread use of various condiments for promotion of appetite and for various presumed therapeutic effects. The common condiments were cinnamon, pepper, and various spices. Sugar was used and the depressant effects of *Hyoscyamus* and *Cannabis indica* were described. There is a poem which was widely used in praise of garlic *(Allium sativum)*, which was applied locally with salt for relief of bites on the skin. There was much interest in aphrodisiacs, and much discussion of antidotes for the bites of venomous snakes. Alcoholic beverages were known and used for relief from tension.

One of the most remarkable of the observations made by the ancient Hindus in regard to the uses of the various plant materials that were tried for food was snakeroot. This was recommended for relief of frenzy or mania. This plant was named *Rauwolfia* in honor of the European botanist who first described it. It has been studied particularly by Indian and Swiss chemists and from it has been isolated a number of indole alkaloids, including reserpine and yohimbine. Currently reserpine is widely used as a mild tranquilizing agent. It is also a useful tool in experimental pharmacology. It is possible that knowledge of the serpent root was brought from India to the Greek world during that conquest of Alexander the Great since serpent root as an agent for the treatment of mania was described by Dioscorides, the surgeon in the armies of Nero. *A survey of Hindu Medicine* (Baltimore, Johns Hopkins Press, 1948) was made by Henry A. Zimmer (1890-1943).

In his excellent compilation, *Indigenous Drugs of India: Their Medical and Economic Aspects* (Calcutta, The Art Press, 1933), Ram Nath Chopra describes a vast number of native Indian drugs. He points out how many Indian remedies have multiplied without adequate testing but by belief, and how difficult it is to obtain reliable background information regarding the indigenous use of these many drugs. Among the drugs which are widely used, probably from antiquity, are *Hydnocarpus wightiana* for leprosy; *Calycopteris floribunda* (Chempulli) as an anthelmintic and laxative, which may contain santonin; *Eclipta prostata* (Babri) as a cholagogue; *Boerahavia defusa* (Punarnava) as a diuretic; *Holarrhena antidysenterica* (Kurchi) and *Bombax malabaricum* (Simul), which probably contained tannin, for dysentery; *Alstonia scholaris* (Chatim), containing the alkaloid ditamine, for malaria, and *Cida cardifolia* (Bala) in diseases of the nervous system and for paralysis.

Other natively used Indian drugs which might be appropriate for investigation are *Adhatoda vasica* (Bakas) as an expectorant and as a useful asthma drug; *Melia azadirichta* (Nim) for relief of fever, *Saraca indica* (Asoka) in menorrhagia; *Terminia arjuna* as a cardiac tonic; *Balsamodendron mukul* (Gugal) as an antirheumatic agent; *Butea frondosa* as an anthelmintic for round worms; *Beganum harmala* (Aspand) as an antiasthmatic and agent for relief of fever; *Saussurea lappa* (Kut) as an aphrodesiac and cardiac stimulant; *Aegle marmels* (Bael), *Plantago ovato* and *Ailiathus malabarica* (Ood) in chronic diarrhea and dysentery; *Herpestes monniera*, (Safed chamni) in hysteria and epilepsy, and the seeds of Bsoralaa corylafolia (Babchi) in leukoderma.

As Chopra indicates, Hindu drugs are many in number and varied in character and the identification of them remains a prime difficulty. He says "No amount of verbal description of these drugs as given in the books will enable the botanist to identify some plants and parts which even in themselves do not invariably present the same characteristics. The result is that there has been a great deal of confusion; many drugs are being sold under various names, different drugs under the same name." He lists eighty-seven plant drugs growing in India from *Acacia arabica* to *Zinzibar officinale*. Many of them are of great antiquity, such as aconite, amygdalin, tragacanth, belladonna, myrrh, mustard, tea, caroway, senna, camphor, cinnamon, colocynth, colchicum, coriander, croton, datura, fennel, gentian, asafetida, juniper, quassia, anise, castor-beans, and viburnum. Many others have been introduced, such as digitalis, ephedra, cacao, ipecac, and nux vomica.

The ancient Hindu drug lore was extensive, but it was not well codified. The various crude drugs were usually simply named in some prescription recommended for some diseased condition or for the relief of some symptom. There may be other useful drugs to be found in the old Indian medical literature, in addition to the isolation of reserpine from snake-root. The observational skill of people of ancient cultures was great in respect to what the plants in their environment could well be used for. Careful study of the recommended drug uses in ancient writings could result in finding agents capable of modern scientific investigation and application.

Sumerian Drugs

In old times the area between the Tigris and Euphrates rivers was well watered and fertile. Here people first seemed to have been able to give up some of their primitive hunting habits and to learn to grow food by cultivation. It was in this area that Emmer wheat *(Triticum dicorcum)* was cultivated. Wild barley *(Hordeum spontaneum)* was also domesticated.

The development of agriculture depends upon close observation of those naturally occurring fruits, vegetables, and grains which may be eaten for food, and it also implies recognition of the ways by which they might be stored so as to provide seed for future crops. In this process many plant materials were discovered which might be used for the alleviation of symptoms of disease.

The medical practices of the peoples in Sumeria were highly developed. In the middle of the nineteenth century, a great library of some thirty thousand clay tablets was discovered in a mound near the site of Ninevah, which had been brought together by Ashurbanipal of Assyria (568-626 BC). Some eight hundred medical tablets have been deciphered, particularly by Morris Jastrow *(Proc R Soc Med, 7:109-176, 1914)*. These indicate that diagnosis was carried out by inspection with the development of a special terminology and that prognosis was indicated particularly by augury of livers at sacrifice, as well as by astrological signs. The etiology was largely demonical. Therapy was ritualistic and many plant remedies were used.

Over one hundred drugs were used, and most of them have been identified as the common plant, animal and mineral materials indigenous to the area. There were two classes of drugs, *shammu* and *abnu,* which Jastrow thinks refer to plant materials on the one hand and mineral materials on the other.

Rheumatism, cardiac disease, stomach troubles, and eye diseases are described in the clay tablets with various remedies recommended. R. C. Thompson has discussed them in his *Assyrian Medical Texts, An Assyrian Herbal* (London, 1926). He indicates that there may have been clinical concepts such as night blindness, *(sin-lurma),* gonorrhea *(musu),* paralysis *(misittu),* scabies *(ikkitic),* and epilepsy *(bennu).*

The Sumerians developed a high degree of specialization in medical practice and had a clear recognition of not only pharmacists and dentists, but also specialists for almost each part of the body. A joke of the period relates how one doctor asks another, "What is your specialty?" to which the reply was "Eyes," to which another question was asked, "Which eye?"

The practice of medicine seems to have been well exploited and was regulated legally. The Code of Hammerabi (2250 BC) includes some fifteen sections describing the penalties for malpractice. These are based on the principle of "an eye for an eye." These constitute the first examples of social regulation of medical practice.

The god of healing was Nineb; he is reputed to have made lists of drugs of plant, animal and insect origin. Many varieties of insects are described and protection was afforded against them with fly traps. The Sumerians knew well how to brew beer, a technical achievement utilizing principles of pharmacy. They also recognized the contagiousness of leprosy and began the strict regulations against it. However, the term *leprosy* might refer to almost any skin disorder.

Sumerian medicine was closely associated with Persian medicine as with Jewish medicine. The Persians seemed simply to have taken over the Sumerian medical practice; many Chinese drugs were also used.

The principal sources of knowledge of Jewish medicine are, of course, the Bible and the Talmud. Disease was considered to be an expression of divine displeasure, and the priests acted as hygienic police. However, priests did not act as physicians. Hyssop was widely used as an agent of catharsis or purification.

One of the major and lasting achievements of the Babylonians was to devise a system of measuring time which is universally used throughout the civilized world today. This important accomplishment similar to the Egyptian success in devising standards for measuring space was part of an effort to relate ourselves to our environment. We are familiar with ourselves both in space and time, and our methods of measuring either space or time are related to our own bodies. The measurement of time became important later in regard to the administration of drugs.

The natural division into day and night was subdivided in each case into twelve equal parts. This was due to the fact that the Babylonians used a duodecimal system of numerical notation. With the method then of counting sets of twelves with reference to the five fingers of the hand, they could handle sixty as a convenient unit. By dividing each one of the twelve parts of day and night, the hours into sixty minutes, and each of these into sixty seconds, they found that they had reached a time interval which is just about the most regular and constant in our own bodies, namely, the heartbeat.

When the ancient Sumerians looked at the skies, they noted that there were seven bodies in the sky that changed their position with reference to the rest. These are the sun, moon, and the five planets which we call Mercury, Mars, Jupiter, Saturn, and Venus. It is obvious that the sun has great influence upon events on the earth.

It was felt that the moon is also highly significant. The moon in ancient cultures was felt in many ways to be superior to the sun, since it can be seen often both at daytime and at night and it changes its shape and form in a regular systematic way. The coincidence of the phases of the moon with the female menstrual cycle was considered to be particularly significant. The moon was the object of worship in all matriarchal primitive societies. In order to be sure that the favor of these heavenly bodies would be obtained, one day in turn was set aside as sacred to each. Sunday, Monday, and so on, for each of these heavenly bodies established the week. Four of these weeks would coincide with the phases of the moon. This established the month, or lunar year.

In primitive societies, this month was the important time measurement and was the convenient method of measuring long times. There is clear evidence, as in the fifth chapter of Genesis, that it was used to estimate the duration of people's lives. In the Book of the Sons of Adam, with the extraordinary number of years of the patriarchs, one will find, if one divides the numbers given by thirteen, which is the number of lunar cycles in a solar year, that these great patriarchs were simply good old men. Methuselah, for example, who was reputed to have lived 969 years, turns out to have been an ordinary old man of 74. That *was* old for those days.

The solar year originally had thirteen lunar months. This provided 364 days, with one left over, which didn't count, and thus became a universal day of license and privilege. Later in an effort to be able to divide the seasons more effectively, a twelve month year was established.

These methods of estimating time became of great importance later in regard to all aspects of living, and were commonplace even through our Middle Ages in the administration of drugs. The procession of the equinoxes, together with the much longer cycle of the ecliptic, established the significance of the constellations in the skies and gave the background to the importance of the zodiac. It is amazing that faith in the influence of heavenly bodies on earthly affairs continues to the present day and is manifest in the wide interest given still to astrology.

Astrological methods were associated with the characteristics of drugs of various sorts. They were used, in an intricate system, to regulate the choice of various drugs for various conditions and to regulate the times of administration of those drugs.

The widespread observational skill of ancient peoples with respect to time measurement is indicated from the amazing character of Stonehenge, and even at the observatory at Uxmal in the old Mayan flatland. The priests regulated the routine activities of their peoples by their determination of the solstices, equinoxes, lunar phases and eclipses.

Peoples have always been in awe of the strange and unknown. Furthermore glimpses of understanding of the infinity of time and space gave a feeling of exaltation. This was furthered in antiquity by ritualistic and social use of intoxicating drugs. Beers were especially well developed in the Babylonian area. Hemp *(Cannabis indica)* was well known as an agent to produce ecstasy and exaltation. It also was recognized as a minor pain relieving agent. Beers probably were laced with preparations of hemp in order to produce hallucinatory effects in connection with ritualistic affairs thus giving all participants a feeling of exaltation and awe.

These matters were carefully regulated by the priesthood. The rituals were established to assure fertility of flocks and fields as well as fertility of families. Many of the rites which survived had first developed in connection with matriarchal cultures.

Of course there must have been abuses of the intoxicating agents, quite as there is now. The story of the drunken Noah confirms this suggestion. Certainly there was abuse also in the use of hemp. The resin from the flowering tops of female plants is highly potent and was known as hashish or bhang. In ancient Persia a group of hashish addicts were accustomed to use the drugs in considerable amounts when gathered together for ritual, and under these circumstances would often go berserk and engage in acts of violence. The word *assassin* is derived from the word *hashish*.

It is remarkable that the social problems associated with *Cannabis indica* still remain with us. Marijuana, which is causing so much current discussion in the United States, is the dried leaves of *Cannabis indica,* which are smoked. The amount of the cannabinols contained in the leaves is much less than that which is contained in the resin-forming hashish. However, enough is absorbed on smoking to give a kick. Perhaps as much harm can be done from smoking joints of marijuana with respect to the possibility of lung cancer as could ever occur from the smoking of tobacco cigarettes. Usually the marijuana smoker inhales deeply, in order to get as much effect as possible.

Two of the common problem drugs of our times were also problem drugs thousands of years ago. The alcoholic beverages have been gradually brought under some degree of social control, but most attempts at legal control of *Cannabis* have not worked satisfactorily. These same problems continue to exist with respect to other mind-moving drugs.

One of the many drugs used for hallucinatory effects in the ancient Sumerian area was the hallucinating mushroom; it, again, has come recently into prominence. The skill required for identifying hallucinating mushrooms from edible or toxic mushrooms was highly developed among the Middle Eastern peoples. Active agents affecting the autonomic and central nervous systems are found in *Amanita muscaria,* as well as in *Amanita pantherina.* There are also indole derivatives found in such mushrooms, e.g. dimethyl-5-hydroxy-tryptamine, which also is in the skins of poisonous toads. It is Howard Fabing's opinion (*Sci Month, 83*:232-237, 1956) that it was the hallucinogenic mushrooms which were responsible for the reported berserkgang of the wild Vikings of the tenth century, and of the widely noted debaucheries of the Siberian Kamchatka tribes, who, in order to "prolong the festivities," made use of the fact that the stimulant is excreted by the kidneys. These mushrooms, as well as *Pantheolus campanulatus,* have been popularly described by Gordon and Valentina Wasson and noted more scientifically by Francisco Guerra and H. Olivera (*Las Plantas Fantasticas de Mexico,* Mexico City, 1954). The mushroom cult of the ancient matriarchies has been well discussed by the English poet, Robert Graves. The hallucinating mushrooms seem to have been widely used in the Eastern Mediterranean in the cult mysteries to give visions of paradise.

It is also likely that some of the extraordinary agents derived from poppy, *Papaver somniferum,* were first observed in the Mesopotamian area. Poppy seed was widely used as a condiment. There is no drug activity in the leaves, fruit, root, or any other part of the plant. However, if the unripe seed capsule is incised, a white juice will exude, which on drying, gives many reasonable drug effects. This is opium. Although this was first mentioned by Scribonius Largus in the first part of our era (*De compositione medicamentorum,* Cratander, Basel, 1529, page 128) there is strong probability that opium was developed much earlier in the Mesopotamian area.

To have discovered opium is an extraordinary instance of the amazing skill of native peoples to find materials in their surroundings which have significant drug effects. Opium is the dried latex of the unripe seed capsules of *Papaver somniferum.* The alkaloids which are characteristic of opium are formed only as the latex dries. The custom is for workmen to move with three-pronged knives through poppy fields in the early evening and cut the unripe seed capsules. The latex exudes and dries overnight. In the morning the men scrape the dried latex off the capsules and collect it in bags. This is opium. This is the material that is a significant sleep-producing agent and also an important pain relieving material.

From the Mesopotamian area, opium probably spread to other

parts of the world. Actually it was not introduced into China until much later. In the nineteenth century, Britain, seeking an outlet for opium production from India, forced the Chinese through the Opium War to import the drug and to use and abuse it. Opium as such was not described in either the ancient clay tablets of the Mesopotamians nor in the early Egyptian medical papyri. It apparently did not come into common use until the beginning of our era.

It is thus clear that the Mesopotamians contributed very significantly to drug lore and to the recognition of indigenous materials that could be used effectively as drugs. In all of this there is evidence of practical reasoning with appropriate uses for drugs, whose properties had been discovered, for the alleviation of the symptoms that various patients might present.

A great deal of Hebraic medicine was derived from the Babylonians as a result of the Babylonian Captivity. However, much Jewish medicine also came from Egypt as a result of the Egyptian Captivity. Much of this is well described by Fielding Garrison (1870-1935) in his always brilliantly written *History of Medicine* (Philadelphia, 4th ed., 1929).

The medical observations of the ancient Hebrews as recorded in the Old Testament are remarkable. Circumcision is a considerable operation, and in its ritual, stone knives were often used. Wounds were dressed, as was the case generally at the time, with wine, oil and soothing gums. An outstanding feature of Hebraic medicine was the careful dietary regiment and the detailed code of ritual hygiene and cult cleanliness. Washing to keep clean was a luxury in arid regions where water was rare.

It is likely that skin lesions were common. Desert sores from dust and dirt might have been confused with leprosy *(Zaraath)*. The healing of Naaman by washing seven times in Jordan was no miracle, but probably the washing away of the dirt that had caused the desert sores. Garrison calls attention to the dangers of speculating about uncertain details in antiquity, calling attention to the point, well known to mathematicians, "that the inherent probability of any occurrence tends the closer to zero the further we get from it, and that the effect of any event tends to die out asymptotically in indefinite or infinite time."

The Jewish Talmud began to accumulate during the Babylonian Captivity around the sixth century BC but was put in its present form much later. The Jewish ritualistic laws governing general hygienic conditions are certainly the beginning of medical jurisprudence. Significantly among the Hebrew the flesh of diseased or injured animals was always considered unfit for food, and the postmortem examinations of slaughtered animals, for the purpose of determining what was *kosher,* tended to give information on pathological conditions that were not known to other peoples. The Jews used veno-section and leeches for removal of foul blood. They devised a sleeping potion *(Samme de shinda)* for pain relief in connection with surgical operations. There is no evidence, however, that this potion contained opium. It may have been hemp.

It is interesting that there were no significant Jewish physicians until the Middle Ages, nor was there any particular specialized medical education among the Jewish people. Nevertheless, there was a high degree of compliance with the standards established by these hygienic laws. Harry Friedenwald (1864-1950) has well discussed *The Jews and Medicine* (Baltimore, Johns Hopkins Press, 1944, 2 volumes).

Altogether the significance of the Mesopotamian peoples in regard to health affairs was great. There probably was considerable interchange along trade routes with India and Egypt, and this probably became extended later to places as far distant as China. Certainly the eastern Mediterranean was greatly influenced in its health affairs by the Mesopotamian area. However, the major influence on the developing Greek world came from Egypt.

Egyptian Drug Codification

Egypt is an area of startling regularity and uniformity. It is an area almost without rain, surrounded by seas and deserts so that it enjoyed a long period of relative peace and quietness. Life in ancient Egypt must have gone on easily and regularly, with a relative abundance of food. The regularity of the annual overflow of the Nile set the pace for the regularity of living. It also was responsible for the necessity of working out standards of measurement for land, which were again developed on the basis of referring our own bodies to our surroundings.

It was necessary, after the annual late summer flood, to re-establish the boundaries of fields in order to prepare for sowing. The old Egyptain method of notation was by doubling or halving. For linear measurement one started with one's finger. Doubling this would be two fingers, but doubling two fingers would give a hand. Doubling a hand gives a span, and doubling a span gives a cubit (knuckles to elbow) and doubling a cubit gives an arm or yard, while doubling an arm gives a fathom.

The Egyptian measurement of food and drugs again originated with reference to our own bodies. One started with a mouthful, a *ro,* the hieroglyph that was a symbol looking like a mouth which developed into the spoon. I have examined old Egyptian wooden and ivory spoons in various museums around the world, and I have found that they all measure about 14 to 15 mls. This then is the common mouthful, two of which gives a handful.

When this form of volume measurement was extended through the Greek-Roman and medieval world into England, it acquired names which are still commonplace with us. The handful is an ounce, and probably originally was a jigger. Two handfuls make a jack. Two jacks are a jill. Two jills are a jug or a pint. While two pints are a quart (a quarter of a gallon), two quarts are a pottle; two pottles are a gallon, and two gallons are a pail. Two pails are a peck; two pecks are a bushel; two bushels are a strike. Two strikes are a coomb; two coombs are a sack; two sacks are a barrel; two barrels are a hogshead, and so on to a tun which is still used for the storage of wines, even in California! It is amazing how the old Egyptian standards for measurement still survive. The liquid measurements were used with respect to the careful instructions for the administration of drugs.

Among the ancient Egyptians, the pharmacists were the skilled specialists in collecting, classifying, analyzing, preparing, and preserving of plant, animal and mineral materials for medical use. They were the ones that were called upon by physicians to make drug preparations, and they did so with responsibility and care.

Drugs were administered in ancient Egypt by volume. Nevertheless, the old Egyptians had already gotten the idea of weight by comparing, say, a handful of kernels of wheat with a handful of gold dust. They do not heft the same. From the movement up and down of the hands in comparing the weights of a handful of gold dust or a handful of wheat kernels must have come the idea for a pan balance. At any rate, pan balances of wood and ivory from old Egypt have been found and carbon dated as early as 3000 BC. The standard of weight was a kernel of wheat. This is remarkably constant and has survived as the grain into our own time.

Our knowledge of old Egyptian drugs comes from the records preserved from antiquity. These are the medical papyri. The original Egyptian recordings were the hieroglyphs made into pictographs or ideographs carved on stone. Later it was found that one could split papyrus reeds and weave them together in a mat, pounding this underwater on a flat stone, drying it, and obtaining a sheet of brown paper. These sheets were about the size of the typewriter paper we use now. They would be written upon by inks prepared from oil with soot or red materials and written from right to left using a split papyrus reed as a stylus. This shorthand form of writing the ideographs or hieroglyphics was called hieratic. The major old Egyptian medical papyri are hieratic writings which were compiled from the period around 2000 BC to 1200 BC. In each instance known, they were probably copied from much older originals. In some instances, these have been estimated to have been at least 3000 BC, to judge from the character of the terminology which was already archaic when the copies were being made, so that the scribe had to explain the meaning of these archaic terms.

There are eight major medical papyri extant from old Egypt. These eight major medical papyri have now been carefully analyzed by the famed Egyptologist, Hermann Grapow. The Kahun papyrus deals chiefly with veterinary medicine but indicates also the examination of women for uterine conditions and signs of pregnancy, with prescriptions made of plant materials and milk.

An amazing teaching document is the Edwin Smith papyrus

(Chicago, University of Chicago Press, 1930, 2 volumes, facsimile and commentary). It was studied carefully by James H. Breasted (1865-1935) of Chicago. It is systematically organized. This is startling in so ancient a medical treatise. Some forty-eight typical cases are given. These are accidental injuries that might have been encountered by individuals in fighting or building. The type cases are presented from the top of the head down through the body. The document is incomplete with the scribe stopping in the middle of a word in the middle of a sentence dealing with an injury to the middle of the back. On the rear of the document are some cosmetic recipes.

The case histories of the Smith papyrus are organized in remarkably clear-cut manner. The title is given in red ink and the text opens with a description of the examination of a patient and what may be found. From this a diagnosis is given. Then there is a prognosis. If the prognosis is favorable, a treatment is recommended. This all has the character of intellectual organization still utilized in medical practice. It is rather astonishing that the ancient Egyptians could have had enough records of similar injuries to have classified them, analyzed them, and systematized information on their appropriate management.

The Ebers medical papyrus is a similar document dealing with medical rather than surgical conditions. It was found by Georg Ebers (1837-1898) and reproduced by him in 1875. An English translation was made by the Danish general practitioner B. Ebbell in 1937. The papyrus seems to be a complete document in 108 hieratic columns, wrongly numbered 110. The material seems to have been brought together from a number of separate sources. It proceeds with many hundreds of recipes classified rather loosely in accordance with the disease states to be treated. There are some cases in which the material is organized by title, examination, diagnosis, prognosis, and treatment.

There are some 829 prescriptions in the document with little duplication. Since it deals with medical conditions where the cause is often obscure, there is not the same clarity of definition of cause as would be possible in a surgical writing, in which the cause of the injury is usually obvious. It is remarkable that there is so little indication of magic and supernaturalism in the text.

It is generally agreed that the Smith and Ebers papyri were designed to be texts for study and training. The Hearst medical papyrus, written during the great eighteenth dynasty, at about the same time as the Ebers, is different. It is a practicing physician's formulary. While there is evidence that there was specialism in medical practice among the old Egyptians, there must have been general practice in the rural areas. It may well have been that some general practitioner from the country, coming into one of the large cites for some purpose, employed a scribe to collect for him a series of prescriptions relating to various disease conditions in which he might have been interested. The haphazard organization of the Hearst medical papyrus suggests that this may have been the situation.

The seventeen sheets of the Hearst Medical Papyrus are among the prized possessions of the University of California. They are preserved in the Anthropology Museum in Berkeley. They have been translated and annotated by Henry Lutz, Sanford Larkey (1898-1969) and myself.

The beginning and ending of the Hearst medical papyrus are frayed and thus incomplete. It was first described in 1905 by George Reisner (1867-1942), to whom it was given when he led the Phoebe Apperson Hearst expedition to Egypt in 1899. It has some 255 prescriptions for a variety of conditions together with recitals designed to promote accuracy and care on the part of the physician or pharmacist in measuring drugs.

The Erman document deals largely with childbirth and diseases of children. There are only two prescriptions recommending simple drugs for an unknown disease of infancy. The London and Berlin medical papyri are similar to each other and were probably written at the end of the eighteenth dynasty, around 1350 BC. These are poorly organized physicians' formularies and contain much of the same material that is to be found in Hearst. The Berlin papyrus contains some two hundred recipes, while the London document has only sixty-one. Like the Hearst medical papyrus, both the Berlin and the London papyri were probably copied from parts of older documents. There is duplication of

TABLE I
THE CHIEF EGYPTIAN MEDICAL PAPYRI

Name & Date	Location	Condition	Contents	References
Kahun 1900 B.C.	London	Framentary, 3 sheets	Unorganized, on women's diseases and pregnancy and veterinary conditions	Griffith, 1898
Edwin Smith 1600 B.C.	New York City	Unfinished, 17 columns	Well organized surgical text; 48 typical cases; cosmetics recipes on verso	Breasted, 130
Ebers 1550 B.C.	Leipzig	Complete in 108 columns (numbered 110)	Medical texts; some 800 recipes classified by diseases; few "cases" anatomical monographs	Ebers, 1875; Wrezinski, 1913; Ebbell, 1937
Hearst 1550 B.C.	Berkeley	Incomplete, 18 columns	Poorly organized practitioner's recipe book with some 260 recipes; an early formulary	Reisner, 1905; Wrezinski, 1912; Lutz, Larkey, Leake, 1939
Erman 1550 B.C.	Berlin	9 columns, 6 on verso	Popular charms for childbirth & care of infants; two prescriptions	Erman, 1901
London 1350 B.C.	London	Fragmentary, 19 columns	Recipe book with recitals	Wreszinski, 1912
Berlin 1350 B.C.	Berlin	22 columns, 3 on verso	Recipes, recitals, signs of pregnancy	Wreszinski, 1909
Chester Beatty 1200 B.C.	London	Incomplete, 8 columns	Formulary for anal diseases, 1 case report	Jonckheere, 1947

prescriptions in the Ebers, Hearst, Berlin, and London papyri. This indicates the extent of the considerable degree of conventionalized drug lore among the ancient Egyptians, which was codified into recommended prescriptions for clinical use.

The various diseases described in the old Egyptian medical papyri are common urinary disorders, fevers, ailments of the heart or stomach, various skin involvements including ulcers, contusions, tumors, orthopedic conditions including pains in bones, joints and muscles (probably rheumatic), cosmetic recipes for skin, head, hair, teeth and eyes, and recitals for the use of the physicians or pharmacists in promoting accuracy in drug measurement. The latter involved what has become a common symbol of Egypt, often associated with magic properties, the "Horus eye." Actually the diagrammatic arrangement of this symbol was simply to provide a reminder of a conversion system in measurement that was necessary in restoring the old system of measurement after a new one had been introduced during the Hyksos invasion (G. Müller, *Ztschr Aegypt Spr, 48*:99-106, 1911). It is significant that 80 percent of the remedies prescribed in the Ebers papyrus for oral administration are quantitated. On the other hand, for cutaneous disorders, treated by local application, only about a third are to be measured.

Of the drugs used by the ancient Egyptians, numbering some two hundred, most are plant, animal and mineral materials found in the environment which probably had been tried for food in some way or other. As the effects of ingesting these materials were noted, those that would cause purgation, for example, were recommended if constipation existed. There are many prescriptions for purging the body. These recommended a variety of vegetable laxatives, such as figs, senna, bitter gourd, and acacia, probably for bulk. The general theory of disease referred to the *whd*, the putrifying material within the body which was thought to cause fermentation, decomposition, decay, and death. This later became the *materia peccans* referred to by medieval writers. It was whatever foul stuff may accumulate in the body that was to be driven out. It probably was this etiological factor which led to such prominence for the use of purgative agents. The major effort of the Egyptian physicians seems to have been directed toward removing *whd* which was thought to be responsible for putrefaction and death.

Many carminative drugs appear as ingredients in the Egyptian medical papyri, including anise, coriander, cumin, and poppy and sesame seeds. These all have some effect in promoting appetite. Barley, beans, peas, and wheat are used in prescriptions for flours for external applications to make poultices for soothing or mild astringent effects. Cinnamon seems to have been introduced from eastern shores and was also used for carminative purposes.

Garlic and leek are recommended for local applications to reduce skin irritations from insect bites. These agents have mild astringent and antiseptic action. Juniper berries have long had a reputation for mild diuretic action. They are frequently recommended in the Egyptian medical papyri for expelling fluid accumulations. Dates are also recommended for this purpose. Castor plant petals or leaves are recommended for prescriptions in promoting urination. Castor oil does not seem to have been recognized as a purgative agent. At any rate, it does not occur as such in the prescriptions.

Locally applied astringent antiseptics were frankincense, gum and myrrh. Some mineral materials such as natron, or sodium carbonate, are specified in prescriptions for local mild astringent antiseptic action. Fat from animal sources is recommended for use in various ointments, and there are some preparations even from fish.

Various beverages are recommended for vechicles for drugs. Beer seems to have been widely used for this purpose. Milk is also employed, and sometimes wine. Honey was frequently used in the Egyptian medical papyri for incorporation in many prescriptions, either for its sweetness or as a binding material. Oil occurs often for carrying drugs for internal administration, and wax was used for binding ingredients into conveniently rolled pills. Soot was sometimes employed, as well as charcoal, clay and even *hot water of the washerman*. These seem to have been used to stop diarrheas.

Some of the ingredients in the Egyptian medical papyri are

not satisfactorily identified. For example, dragon's blood may be either cinnabar (red mercuric sulfide) or it may also be *Resina draconius* from an East Indian palm tree. This confusion regarding dragon's blood persisted in European formularies through medieval to relatively modern times.

One may conclude that the relatively large number of drugs recommended by the old Egyptian physicians for various disease conditions seems to have a rational basis, with sensible applications to disease conditions of the readily observable actions of crude animal, plant and mineral materials occurring in the environment, i.e. materials which must have been noted in the continuous search for food, or as a result of accidental contact. No significant poisonous or toxic agents were recommended, nor were toxic amounts indicated. The various drugs recommended for therapeutic use in the old Egyptian papyri would seem to tend toward beneficial results even as judged by modern knowledge.

Mid-American Medicine

Our knowledge of Middle American drugs comes chiefly from two documents, the *Badianus Codex* and the *Zahagun Codices*. The *Badianus Codex* was written by Martin de la Cruz, a native physician who was a student at one of the Franciscan monasteries in Mexico. The Codex was wrongly named after Juan Badiano, the Mexican scribe at the monastery who prepared a Latin version of the information given in the native Nahuatl in 1552. This manuscript, with beautiful reproductions of medicinal herbs, is in the Vatican Library. An English translation with facsimile of the original was published in 1940 by Emily W. Emmart (*The Badianus Manuscript, Codex Barbareni, Latin 241, Vatican Library, An Aztec Herbal of 1552*, Baltimore, Johns Hopkins Press, 1940). A Spanish version with an analysis was published by Francisco Guerra (*Libellus medicinalibus Indorum Herbis*, Mexico City, Vargas Resay Diario Espanol, 1952).

The *Zahagun Codices* are a group of manuscripts on the early Mexicans written by a Francisco friar, Bernardino de Zahagun (1499-1590), who came early to Mexico and devoted his life to an exhaustive study of the Aztecs. A draft of his Tepepulco work of

1559 gives a list of ailments and their remedies. Later and more extensive writing was translated into English by C. E. Dibble and A. J. O. Anderson (*Florentine Codex, General History of the Things of New Spain,* University of Utah, Santa Fe, 13 volumes, 1950-1963).

These works have been well summarized by Francisco Guerra (*Medical History, 10*:315-338, 1966). Guerra's first-hand knowledge of the country and of the materials with which he has worked gives his opinions significant weight. Furthermore, his analyses are clear and well organized.

Aztec physicians used herbs and applied remedies if they considered the ailment to be of minor significance. On the other hand, if they thought that the diseases were acute, it was customary to use religious rituals in addition to the indigenous materia medica. As Guerra says, the recipes in the native codices resemble the medieval formularies, particularly in their generous use of botanical remedies. There are some mineral and animal materials recommended. Guerra points out that there is no indication of the mode of action of the drugs in the various prescriptions, nor is there any apparent connection between the presumed causes of disease from the virtues, if any, of the ingredients of the prescriptions. There are 251 plants noted in the *Badianus Codex* with 185 pictured in color. Zahagun mentions 123 plant remedies.

The extraordinary number of plant remedies used in Central-America is indicated by Francisco Hernandez (*Rarum medicarum Novae Hispaniae Thesaurus,* V. Mascardi, Roma 1628), in listing something like 1200 medicinal plants. Guerra indicates the soundness of Nahuatl botanical nomenclature in respect to the names of the various plants referring to their physical characteristics or properties or attributes, with clear consistency. It is significant that they recognized the double meaning of drugs, similar to the recognition by the ancient Greeks, of both medicinal and poisonous properties. The drug gardens found by the conquistadors in Tenochitlan aroused their deep admiration. From them the conquerors became acquainted with maize, potatoes, new types of beans, coca, chili, cotton, rubber and tobacco. They found that the Mexicans were using jalap, castor oil, and balsam and sarsaparilla and smilax were introduced particularly for the treatment of syphilis.

Guerra and Hector Olvera have reported on the extensive number of hallucinating drugs used by the Aztecs (*Las plantas fantasticas de Mexico,* Mexico City, Diario Espanol, 1954). This includes the hallucinating mushrooms, *Peyotl,* a cactus containing mescaline, *Ololiuqui,* the morning glory, which contains lysergic acid derivatives, and *Toluah,* which is related to the daturas. The "woman's medicine," *Cihuapatli,* has been found to have oxytocic action. Guerra has further reported on ethnobotanical sources of Mexican phantastica with historical data on ten such agents (*Br J Addict, 62*:111-127, 1967).

With the wide number of diseases rather clearly indicated by the Mayans, as shown by Guerra, there must have been equally effective observational skill in the utilization of various plant remedies for effective therapy. There remains considerable difficulty in the satisfactory identification of the plant remedies used, although it is clear that pharmaceutical skill was involved in the preparation of some of the prescriptions. It was known how to extract, apparently by boiling, and how to prepare effective ointments. Guerra notes that over four hundred Mayan prescriptions have been collected from various sources.

It is clear then that the same conditions existed in Central-America in the development of effective drugs for various purposes, as had occurred in China, India, Mesopotamia, and Egypt. Apparently indigenous peoples everywhere learned, in the process of seeking food, what the actions may be of the various plant, animal and mineral materials in their environment. Usually they tend to employ such materials with reasonableness in the treatment of disease. When a plant is discovered that will cause emesis, it may be recommended for vomiting when there is stomach distress, or when a plant is found that will cause purgation, it is usually recommended for use when an individual is constipated. Although we have no records of the materia medica of the Incas corresponding to that which has been so well studied from Mayan and Aztec sources, it is likely that there was in the high Peruvian culture similar skill in the recognition, preparation and use of indigenous plant, animal and mineral remedies.

Thus, it appears likely that all over the world, indigenous people have learned the medicinal properties of the plant, animal and mineral materials in their environments which are appropriate and satisfactory for medical use. Many are recognized as being useful for internal administration but many also are realized to have local soothing action when applied to the skin. Even though there may not have been any clear or satisfactory theory either of disease or infection, it would seem that experience in itself was sufficient to give a great body of drug lore. In the beginning this was probably passed along verbally, only gradually to be analyzed, systematized, organized, and codified. This, of course, must have taken time. The miracle is that it was done at all. Further, it is astonishing that the drug lore so painstakingly collected has persisted for so long. Indeed in some cases now it has been found to be very worthwhile to examine the native remedies and their native uses from the standpoint of systematic scientific investigation in accordance with modern standards.

* * * * *

Friends help: I wanted something on drug use by the Incas of Peru; it came from Michael Horowitz of the Fitz Hugh Ludlow Library in San Francisco. Recently it issued a full reprint of W. Golden Mortimer's *History of Coca: the "Divine Plant" of the Incas* (1974, 576 pp.). This is a broad survey of coca and cocaine, originally published in 1901, and always a rare item. Mortimer shows how Incas overcame the hardships of life in the Andes by chewing coca leaves, with a little lime. This relieved fatigue and gave exhileration, without apparent harm. Coca leaves, the crude drug, may be better than its alkaloid, cocaine, as a tonic and stimulant. We may continue to learn from folk-lore!

CHAPTER 4

GRAECO-ROMAN MEDICINE

Poisons and medicine are oftentimes that same substance given with different intents.

PETER M. LATHAM (1789-1875)

THE TRANSITIONS FROM ANCIENT Egyptian to Greek medicine have been well documented by J. B. de C. M. Saunders (Lawrence, University of Kansas Press, 1963). Robert O. Steuer and he have also discussed the relations between ancient Egyptian and Cnidian medicine (Berkeley University of California Press, 1959). While this treats the relationship of the etiological concepts of disease between the ancient Egyptian and Greek physicians, it offers an understandable background for the transmission of codified formulary drug lore from ancient Egypt into the Greek world.

We have little material with which to reconstruct the important medical group which centered around Cnidos on the Asia Minor mainland. This school was greatly overshadowed by the preeminence of the group of health professions centering on Kos, across the water from Cnidos. The presumed interrelations of these two groups have been interestingly reconstructed by Wilder Penfield, the great Montreal neurosurgeon, in his brilliant novel, *The Torch*. This is a fictionalized account of the great Coan physician, Hippocrates (460-375 BC). Hippocrates was certainly a great teacher. Even the old plane tree under which he is reputed to have taught in Kos is still thought to be standing.

The various writings ascribed to Hippocrates, however, probably are from the group of which he was clearly the most prominent member. These works have been carefully collated from surviving Greek texts by the great Parisian scholar, Emile Littre (1801-1881). This is a vast work in ten volumes published in Paris between 1839 and 1861. There are two major English translations, one, the two volume Sydenham Society publication in 1849 by Francis Adams (1796-1861) and the other, the London edition of 1923 to 1931 edited by W. H. S. Jones.

The writings of the Hippocratic school show these physicians to have been eminently rational in their approach to medical affairs. Eschewing all magical associations in relation to disease, they even declared, in regard to the sacred disease (epilepsy), that it is no more sacred than any other disease and that it has a natural cause and a satisfactory method of handling it will be evolved. It has taken a long while to fulfill this prophecy, but it is occurring.

The members of the Hippocratic School wrote brilliantly on geographical medicine and on various acute and chronic diseases. They had a high ethical standard and were brilliant in surgery, probably taking their surgical techniques from the earlier Egyptians.

On the other hand, the Hippocratic physicians seem to have little to do with drugs. They recognized that sick people tend to get well regardless of treatment. This principle became the famed *Vis medicatrix naturae* of the later Greco-Romans. It is interesting that periodically this "healing power of nature" must be rediscovered. Currently we are doing so in connection with the placebo effect as observed in double-blind crossover experimental studies on humans with new drugs.

It may be assumed that the Hippocratic physicians used the drug materials already formulated by the Egyptians into recommended prescriptions for various disease states. However, there is no indication that the Hippocratic physicians were much impressed by drugs. Rather they relied upon dietary control, good nutrition, and calm moderate living.

We do not know whether the Hippocratic physicians took over the Egyptian ideas on etiology of disease with special reference to *wdw* (the putrefying principle responsible for illness, malaise, and even death) which is to be expelled from the body whenever possible. The Hippocratic physicians were beginning to take over the humoral pathology which was developing philosophically from Asia Minor and Athenian philosophers.

The four humors were derived from the basic four elements of water (Thales, 639-544 BC), fire or heat (Heraclitus, 566-460 BC), and air and earth (Empedocles, 504-433 BC). The qualities of these elements were moisture from water, heat from fire, cold from air, and dryness from earth. The four humors of the body were derived from combinations of the qualities of the four elements in relation to a scale of life running from the most living toward death: blood (the sanguine temperament, being hot and moist from fire and water); phlegm (phlegmatic temperament, moist and cold from water and air); yellow bile or maybe urine (bilious temperament, hot and dry from earth and fire); and black bile (melancholic temperament, probably from blackwater fever, the terminal stage of malaria, being dry and cold and thus nearest death, from earth and air). Treatment in general consisted in trying to balance these humors by removing excesses or by replenishing deficiencies.

In the replenishing of deficiencies of any one of the humors it was essential to understand the qualities of various foods, or of various medicaments whether plant, animal or mineral in origin. Thus if it were felt that there might be a lack of phlegm, one should eat plenty of seafood, including molluscs, such as oysters and clams, which are moist and cold. Usually, however, physicians could diagnose the difficulty in patients by reference to an excess of one or more of the humors. Thus if it were thought that there might be too much blood, the patient would have blood removed by piercing a vein; if too much phlegm, the individual was purged or vomited; if too much urine, the patient was sweated, and if there might be too much black bile, there was practically nothing that could be done. These drastic treatments of bleeding, purging, vomiting, and sweating were continued well into the early nineteenth century.

A beginning scientific background for the practical affairs of the health professions was provided by Aristotle (384-322 BC); he made careful observations on animals of all sorts and suggested a classification running from the simple to the more complex. He described the parts of animals and studied their generation. His pupil Theophrastus (380-287 BC) classified plants and noted their medicinal properties. This was the beginning of a systematic analysis of remedies on the basis of their individual characteristics, rather than a codification of combinations as in the Egyptian formularies where the drug materials were recommended for treatment.

Greek medicine was widely disseminated through the Roman Empire by Greek physicians, who often were slaves. Their high intellectual standard, nevertheless, commanded the respect of their masters, and frequently they were freed and enjoyed a relatively high social status. The Romans themselves, however, held to the standard of high personal hygiene. It was considered the responsibility of the father of a family to keep all members of the family in good physical condition. This tendency was greatly exemplified by that urbane encylopedist, Celsus, who is the only one of the great Greco-Roman medical writers to use Latin.

The eight books of Celsus are a compendium of medical practice, apparently designed for the benefit of families who wished to keep themselves in good physical condition. There are excellent accounts of surgical procedures and full accounts of various diseases, both acute and chronic, and of various pathological conditions, including the famed reference to the signs of inflammation. Celsus goes into great detail with regard to the virtues of various foods and their qualities and thus their usefulness in making up deficiencies of any one of the four humors. Similarly he treats exhaustively drugs of various sorts using those which had already been introduced from Egypt or Sumeria into the Greek world.

There was no social regulation of medical practice in the Greco-Roman world, and thus quackery tended to flourish. Nevertheless, there were clear efforts to bring rational understanding in regard to health practices. One of the most important was devised by Dioscorides, the surgeon who tramped all over the Empire with the armies of Nero. Dioscorides collected all the information he could on drugs that were commonly used. He brought this vast material together in a compilation which is usually given the Latin title, *Materia Medica*. This comprises an account of all the various drugs of which Dioscorides could learn. The important feature about the compilation is its organization. It treats each separate drug by itself. In each case, the drug is discussed from the standpoint of its various names, its sources, how to identify it, how to tell whether or not it has been adulterated, how it is prepared for administration, what it will do, and what it is used for. There may be an occasional comment on its potential toxicity if used in excess.

This is a rational approach. It afforded a standard guide for the identification of drugs and thus may have been a considerable factor in tending to keep quackery and exploitation under control. Certainly it was popular. It is clear that it may have been illustrated from the first.

It would seem that the work of Dioscorides was well illustrated from its inception. The magnificent manuscript of the work of Dioscorides from the fifth century, which is now in Vienna, carries illustrations for each one of the plant materials, so that identification is rendered possible. These illustrations became conventionalized. They seem to have derived from a Greek artist named Krateus. His work was carefully studied by the great medical historian, Charles Singer.

Dioscorides described some six hundred plants. This is about a hundred more than was discussed by Theophrastus. Apparently, around 150 of these plant remedies were already known to the Hippocratic group. Dioscorides divided his work in a qualitative manner from the standpoint of medicinal use rather than from any attempt at botanical arrangement. He seems to have recognized natural families of plants, but his organization deals with pharmaceutical preparations. The first book is concerned with aromatic, gummy, or oily plant products. The second book is concerned with animal products of dietetic and medical value, and with cereals and garden vegetables. The third and fourth books treat medicinal plants and herbs together with medicinal roots, while the fifth book describes vines and wines. The sixth book discusses metals which are used in medicine as well as other types of metallic materials.

These descriptions of Dioscorides were followed for some sixteen centuries and formed the basis for the materia medica of this long period. The Julia Anicia manuscript of Dioscorides, which is in Vienna, has been reproduced in photographic facsimile. This Vienna manuscript dates from around 512 AD and was prepared for the Byzantine princess, Julia Anicia. There is a ninth century manuscript in Paris which also is well illustrated. There is again an illustrated manuscript of Dioscorides in Venice. The Cheltenham manuscript of the tenth century is in the Pierpont Morgan Library in New York. Dioscorides was translated into Latin by the sixth century and was extensively translated and commented upon in the sixteenth century. The Greek text was printed by the Aldus brothers in 1499 and the Mattioli Latin text and commentary appeared in 1554 and went through many editions.

An important English translation of Dioscorides was made by John Goodyear in 1655 and was edited by Robert T. Gunther and published in 1934. John Goodyear was a botanist of Petersfield, who wrote out the entire Greek text of Dioscorides and made an interlinear English translation. This suggests that Dioscorides was known to the great English herbalists of the sixteenth century. Goodyear's book was never printed, but remained for years in the Magdalen College Library in Oxford. The illustrations were taken from the Julia Anicia manuscript and apparently were based upon originals of Krateus, who was an herbalist in his own right. He had been the physician to Mithridates VI (120-63 BC) who was well respected for his knowledge about poisons and antidotes. The potent antidote mithridatum was named for him. Krateus was widely recognized as a competent artist. Charles Singer (1876-1962), the great historian of medicine, has tentatively identified at least eleven plant figures in the Julia Anicia manuscript as derived from Krateus. He thought that of some 345 plants, ninety-three were well characterized, but that some thirty-six were probably fictitious. Gunther agrees that many of the plant figures are hopeless of interpretation.

In the introduction to his work Dioscorides indicated, in writing to his friend Areius, that he had consulted many previous writers about plants, and he directly referred to Krateus as being better versed on useful medicinal roots than others. Dioscorides suggested that a treatise on medicine was necessary and that it would be helpful in affording direction of methods of preparations and of mixtures and even of experiments on diseases, because the knowledge of each separate medicine would enable one to understand what would be expected from it. He suggested that medicinal plants found growing on plains, in forests and shady localities where the wind cannot blow through are, for the most part, the weaker. He also pointed out that in order to recognize plants accurately, one must be trained to follow them from their beginning to their full fruition. He also indicated that most plants will only be good for use for a few years, but that white and black hellebore *(Veratrum album* and *niger)* retain their powers for many years. He pointed out that flowers and sweet scented things should be laid up in dry boxes of lime wood, but that some herbs do well wrapped in papers or leaves for the preservation of their seeds. For moist medicines, he suggested that thicker material, such as glass or horn, would be best and that earthenware might also be used.

He differentiates between pot herbs and sharp herbs and between various kinds of roots. Famed is his description of mandragora, the root of which he indicates may be made into a preparation which will cause some degree of sleepiness and a relief of pain. Mandragora became a favorite ingredient of anesthetic preparations during the Middle Ages. It has a long legendary history in relation to fertility.

The clearcut manner with which Dioscorides described each separate medicinal agent, whether plant, animal or mineral, established the background for later pharmacopeias. The most significant example of a Dioscordian approach to medicinal agents is the important *Merck Index*. Its eighth edition in 1968 includes nearly ten thousand descriptions of individual substances with some 42,000 names of various chemicals and drugs. The *Merck Index* first appeared in 1889. Under Paul G. Strecher and his associates as editor, it is truly an encylopedia of chemicals and drugs.

On the other hand, the most recent example of an effective

formulary along the lines of the old Egyptian medical papyri is the *Merck Manual,* which was in its eighth edition in 1950. This is a volume of over 1500 pages and lists various prescriptions that are recommended for various disease conditions. In this respect it follows the example set by the old Egyptian medical papyri. There is an addition, the *Merck Veterinary Manual,* which is, in 1967, in its third edition. This is a volume of more than 1600 pages and again is arranged on the basis of recommended procedures in connection with various veterinary disorders. The eleventh edition of the *Merck Manual* (1966) has over 1800 pages and is extensively organized with regard to various disease conditions and various methods of diagnosis and treatment. The recommended drug treatment is particulary extensive. From the Dioscordian type of compilation of separate drugs, with particular emphasis on methods of identification, evolved the pharmacopeias which are so characteristic of the sixteenth into the twentieth centuries. The pharmacopeias were primarily established for the purpose of offering members of the health professions guidelines for the identification of drugs and for determining the purity of the drugs that might be used. The United States Pharmacopeia was first established in 1820, and has been revised every ten years. Currently the *United States Pharmacopeia* is not so much a satisfactory guide for the identification of drugs as it is a glossy-legal list of chemical agents and drugs which are agreed upon as being useful for certain purposes. It is by no means a satisfactory reference work for the identification of all the various kinds of chemicals or drugs that members of the health professions may wish to use.

Greek medicine was solidly established in Rome by Aesclepiades of Bithynia who flourished around 125 BC. While he opposed the Hippocratic idea that sickness is due to a disturbance of body humors, he had another idea in which he thought disease was due to a constriction or relaxation of the solid particles of the body. This idea has been revived at various times. While Aesclepiades theoretically might have opposed the Hippocratic notion of the healing power of nature, he did actually practice on the basis of good diet, massage, hydrotherapy, and with sparing medication.

He was a pioneer in the humane treatment of mental disorder. He used wines to promote sleep. His methodical program helped to develop other systems of medical practice, one of which emphasized the importance of airs. This developed into a pneumatism. Most of the great Roman physicians, however, were electics, and committed to no single regimen of therapy.

The possibility of poisoning developed into popular fear during Roman times. Toxic effects of plant, mineral and animal materials must have been recognized in the continuing search for food. It is significant that none of the great codified formularies or prescription writings of China, India, Sumeria, Egypt or Maya recommended potentially poisonous materials. Proposed dosages were generally low.

However, with no knowledge of pathogenic microorganisms, it would be expected that people might often experience vomiting, abdominal pain, and diarrhea, resulting from contaminated foods or drinks, and ascribe the symptoms to deliberate poisoning by some enemy.

Rulers were especially fearful. It is reputed that quasi-experimental toxicology was studied by certain cautious rulers as an outgrowth of Alexandrian ideas of around 200 BC. Mithridates (120-63 BC), King of Pontus, became famed for his efforts to prevent poisoning by developing a universal antidote. As reported by Gilbert Watson in his interesting *Theriac and Mithridatium* (London, Wellcome Historical Medical Library, 1966, 165 pp.), this mithridatium had thirty-five ingredients ranging from anise through pepper to styrax. Celsus quoted it, and this indicates its presumed importance to the Romans. Robert Graves, the brilliant English poet, suggests that the Roman Emperor Claudius (10 BC -54 AD) was poisoned by his wife, Agrippina, by feeding him poisonous mushrooms, amanita phalloides.

As early as the third century BC, Nikander, a priest of Apollo and a physician at Claros in Asia Minor, wrote a poem of 636 hexameter Greek verses on poisons called *Alexiphormaka*, referring to hemlock, aconite, fungi of various sorts, curdled milk, and lead salts. He described symptoms and remedies. The latter were usually purgatives with olive oil as an emetic. This served as a model for many later writings on antidotes, clear into the nineteenth century.

Nikander also wrote a *Theriaka* in 958 hexameter Greek lines dealing with venomous creatures, how to avoid their bites and what to use if bitten. His universal antidote here is the "great century," *Chlora perfoliata,* the leaves of which are crushed to be applied to the wound, and made into a decoction with wine to be drunk. The virtues of this plant are said to have been discovered by Chiron, the Centaur, and teacher of Aesklepios.

As shown by Gilbert Watson, this *Theriaka* of Nikander was probably taken from a third century BC Alexandrian, Apollodorus, who wrote a treatise on venomous creatures. Indeed, by Galen's time there were already many physicians who had written about antidotes for poisons or venomous bites. Galen (131-201 AD) himself wrote several such, including those called Antidotes I, dealing with special theriacs, Antidotes II, concerning collections of over a hundred antidotes, and *Theriake,* a continuance of Antidotes I. Galen refers to the viper's flesh mithridatium of the Cretan Andromachus, physician to Nero, the third century BC Greek physician, Nileus, whose mithridatium already had 58 ingredients, and Apollonius Mus, a physician of the first century BC. Many others are listed by Galen. In general, Galen's lists are similar to those given earlier by Pliny (23-79 AD). For details, one should consult Gilbert Watson's important monograph.

From the standpoint of drugs, Galen, the vigorous physician to Roman patricians in the second century, was especially important. Galen was born in Pergamon, where there was one of the greatest of the Aesklepia. He must have come under the influence of the more rational aspects of medical care at Pergamon early. He is reputed to have treated gladiators, and then after traveling extensively, he settled in Rome. Although he left no satisfactory case records, he nevertheless instituted an elaborate system of drug use. As vegetable simples, this survived to our time in the term, *galenicals.* Galen's *De Simplicibus,* which was written around 180 AD, was the only Greek herbal comparable to that of Dioscorides. It was used extensively by Oribasius (325-403), the physician to Julian the Apostate. Galen described plant, animal and mineral materials used as the drugs in a systematic rational manner, giving sources, methods of identification, qualities with reference to the standard humoral theory, uses and methods of administration. Nothing particularly new was added. Yet it was all given in such an authoritative way that it became a major source of reference for centuries.

Galen was a theorist, but nevertheless performed experiments. His works are a tremendous encyclopedia of the medical knowledge of his time, including nine books on anatomy, seventeen on physiology, six on pathology, fourteen on therapeutics, sixteen on the pulse, and thirty essays on pharmacy. He was a keen clinician, describing aneurysm and different forms of phthisis for which he recommended a milk diet. His prescriptions suggest rational use for opium, wine, honey, hellabore, hyoscyamus, collocynth, turpentine, barley water and grape juice.

Galen started experimental physiology and showed that the arteries contain blood. He indicated the pump power of the heart by showing that blood pulsates between the heart and a ligated artery, but not beyond that. He also showed that an excised heart will beat outside the body.

In general, Galen tried to follow Hippocratic teachings, but was too much of a theorist. He made dogma of the four humors and developed a physiological schema operating on the basis of three types of fluids. Foods, digested in the stewpan of the stomach are converted into chyle, which passes to the liver, where it is formed into the natural spirits which are transmitted by veins to provide nourishment to all parts of the body. Some of these natural spirits pass from the right side of the heart, where they are mixed with air from the lungs, to go by pores in the septum of the heart, into the left ventricle of the heart, where they are made into vital spirits. These are distributed by arteries to all parts of the body for warmth and life. Some of these vital spirits going through the cribiform plate at the base of the brain are made into animal spirits which are transmitted by nerves to all parts of the body for motion. This was a logical scheme and was extended systematically with vast detail. Garrison implies that this elaborate scheme of things is a carryover from Cnidian medicine and has left its mark on textbooks in medicine until relatively recent times.

The physiological scheme of Galen was followed dogmatically until the seventeenth century. Unfortunately, Galen thought that pus formation was an essential feature in the healing of wounds. This idea was widely developed later. Galen's influence was tremendous. He was a clear and voluminous writer and he was considered to be the final authority in medical affairs. Actually he was not as practical as Aretaeus, who lived a little later and followed the Hippocratic example of clear accuracy in describing diseased conditions.

Another considerable Roman writer was Rufus of Ephesus, who lived a century earlier than Trajan and who was a skilled anatomist and clinician. He added several new compounds for therapeutics, one of which was the *hiera,* a purgative containing collocynth.

In the second century AD, Soranus of Ephesus wrote more extensively on obstetrics and pediatrics than other Greco-Roman writers. Soranus' writings on pediatrics contain rational precepts regarding infant nutrition and hygiene and describe rickets. He emphasized balanced nutrition for youngsters.

In the first century AD, Pliny the Elder (23-79 AD) wrote an encyclopedia containing a vast amount of extraordinary information and ideas. Pliny extolled the ideal of individual hygiene and took many cracks at physicians. His writings contain many remarkable ideas about plants and drugs. It is in Pliny that the mandragora juice was referred to as narcotic, and it is in Pliny that various experiments with poisons were described. Much of the plant lore described by Pliny was derived from Theophrastus and the Alexandrians.

Another first century Roman writer was Scribonius Largus, who compiled a *Compositiones Medicorum,* which contains many prescriptions and accounts of many drugs. In the Cratander edition of Scribonius Largus, translated by Guinter of Andernach, there is the first description of opium as given from antiquity. This occurs as Chapter 180 and describes the way by which the juice exudes from the unripe seed capsule and how it is gathered after it is dried for use. It is suggested that it be given in a water emulsion for the purpose of producing sleep and relieving pain.

The Byzantine Compilers

With the gradual decline of the influence of Rome, as Christianity developed in the Near East, Byzantium became the center of the Eastern Empire. This city was founded by Constantine the Great, who had established Christianity as the state religion. His son, Julian, tried to restore pagan worship but failed.

The outstanding physician of this time was Oribasius (325-403 AD). Trained in Pergamon, as was the case with Galen, Oribasius became physician to Julian and was outstanding in compilations of medical information. Julian asked him to get together a summary of the ideas of Galen. This set Oribasius to work and he did expound Galenical ideas in a very successful way. Furthermore, he referred in detail to the works of his predecessor. His encyclopedia of medicine comprised some seventy volumes in the original. Only seventeen of the books remain and these were translated carefully by Johann Baptiste Rosarius (sixteenth century).

One of the most interesting of the manuscripts of Oribasius, with the Latin translation by Rosarius, was published both in the original Greek and in the Latin translation from Moscow in 1808. An epitome of this work was published as a synopsis and became a very popular item. During the Middle Ages, Oribasius' works were widely known and were very influential in establishing the basic nutritional ideas for many years. Oribasius gives detailed discussions on the qualities of various food materials, with respect to their influence in altering the humors of the body and in determining the temperament. While he obtained most of his information from his predecessors, he is remembered for his description of the effects of intimidation of intelligent children by browbeating at the hands of incompetent schoolmasters. The best edition of Oribasius is that given by C.V. Daremberg (1817-1872) which was in six volumes and included the Greek and French. This was published in Paris between 1851 and 1876. The Aldine edition of the *Synopsis* was published in Venice in 1554. Altogether Oribasius was an outstanding figure in the development of our knowledge of drugs in that he analyzed and recorded all the major information on drugs from antiquity.

This he passed on to those who followed him.

In the sixth century Aetius was also a Byzantium court physician. He also reported much on the contributions of his predecessors, but made his clinical descriptions more accurate. He recommended many ointments for surgical application and plasters for counter irritation. As a Christian, he proposed prayers for use with medicaments. The brother of the architect of Sancta Sophia was Alexander of Tralles (525-605). While a Galenist, he had much originality, especially on intestinal worms, which he well described, and on the use of effective vermifuges, such as fern-root, wormwood, chenopodium and santonin, which remained standard until our time. He first recommended rhubarb as a purgative and colchicum for gout. The latter is still used.

Here let it be clear that hind-sight rationalizing may not be justified. The ancient medical and pharmacy writers rarely indicated preference of one drug over another in the many usually recommended for the same purpose. Thus, Alexander of Tralles, in his recommendations for removing worms, includes celery, leek, parsley, garlic, cumin, mint, pomegranate pips, cress, castor oil, walnuts, cabbage seeds in olive oil with rue and portulaca, as well as enemas of cedar oil and camomile. Long experience, trial and statistical success, led gradually to the recognition in the nineteenth century that only fern-root, wormwood, chenopodium and santonin are real anthelmintics.

The last of the great Byzantine compilers was Paul of Aegina (625-690). With little originality except in surgery, his seven books on medical practice are important chiefly for the extensive commentary upon them in the English translation by the keen Scottish general practitioner, Francis Adams (1796-1861), which was published in three volumes by the Sydenham Society of London in 1834-1847. This commentary gives references to Greco-Roman Muslim and medieval medical writers on every drug and food-stuff mentioned. It is a rich volume of drug information and a brilliant achievement of classical scholarship. It is interesting that the Byzantine medical literature included a veterinary treatise, with prescriptions for farm animals, by Publius Vegetius of the fifth century.

CHAPTER 5

THE MUSLIM DRUG INNOVATIONS

> Give me to drink mandragora....
> That I might sleep.
>
> WILLIAM SHAKESPEARE (1564-1616)
> *Antony and Cleopatra,* I, v.

IT IS NO MORE APPROPRIATE to refer to Muslim medicine as Arabic medicine than it would be to call medieval European medicine Latin medicine. Most Muslim medical writings, except some Hebraic tracts, were written in Arabic, quite as most medieval European medical treatises were written in Latin. Those were the common scholarly languages for the Mohammedan and Christian worlds, respectively.

Muslim medicine carried forward the Graeco-Roman professional medical tradition, although popularly many older Sumerian, Egyptian and Coptic medical practices persisted. The relatively high intellectual standards of the Muslims tended, however, to reduce superstitions and magical practices to a minimum. Yet, astrology, as developed by the ancient Babylonians, continued to be studied by professional physicians and public alike.

Graeco-Roman medicine came into the Muslim world by way of the Nestorian sect of Arians, who had a considerable school at Gondisapor in Persia. The followers of Bishop Arius had been driven from the established church as heretics, following the Council of Nicea in 325 AD. They claimed Jesus was no more divine than any other person and that there is only one God. Nestorius, a patriarch of Constantinople in 428 AD, went on to insist that Mary was the mother of Jesus, but not mother of God.

The Nestorians first taught at Edessa in Mesopotamia, where there was an excellent hospital, but fled to Persia in 489. They probably first translated the Graeco-Roman medical classic into Persian, for practical use. The Persian medically trained physicians became the major medical teachers, after the rise of the Baghdad Caliphate around 749. Some even penetrated as far east as India and China.

Mohammed (570-632) was a fiery fanatic Arian who so inflamed his followers that they had conquered Asia Minor, North Africa, and Spain within a couple of centuries after his death. The vigor of the effort continued in a magnificent cultural development centering in Baghdad in the east, in Kairouan in North Africa, and in Cordoba in Spain.

The Islamic contributions to protopharmacology were considerable. The chief developments were in such pharmaceutical inventions as syrups for respiratory afflictions, distillation with special reference to obtaining medicinal concentrates from beer and wines, and, in therapy, by introducing mercurial ointments as specifically curative for skin eruptions, perhaps including large pox.

As Sleim Ammar puts it in his well organized and informative *En Souvenir de la Médicine Arabe* (Bascone & Muscat, Timis, 1965, 209 pp.) there were three periods in Muslim medicine: 1) assimilation and translation of Graeco-Roman classics under the Nestorians at Gandisapor in Persia; 2) modification of classic concepts as a result of Muslim experience, with incorporation of Alexandrian traditions from the eighth to the thirteenth centuries, and 3) the diffusion of the Arabic language medical tradition to Western Europe via Salerno and Montpelier.

By 887 there was already a medical training center with hospital in Kairouan, when Isaac Ibn Omrane wrote on simple medicaments, mostly plant preparations and wines. He took his material from Galen and condensed it for teaching effectiveness. Isaac Ibn Soleiman, also probably Jewish, wrote in the tenth century on drugs and foods, and prepared a treatise on weights and measures used in pharmacy. Zad el Moucafir, or Viatique, in the eleventh century wrote on simple and compound drugs and

The Muslim Drug Innovations

on poisons. In the Grand Mosque of Tunis is a fourteenth century manuscript of Mohammed Eccherif Essakaly comprising twenty-five chapters of pharmaceutical information on the composition, preparation, preservation and indications for the use of tablets, powders, pills, electuaries, collyria, suppositories, syrups, tinctures, plasters and other technical pharmacy products.

In his clear manner, Ammar divides the development of the health professions in the Eastern Caliphate, chiefly medicine and pharmacy, into a theocratic period, the Ommeiadic time, and the Abbessiche era, which as it declined, led to much productive originality. The theocratic period was dominated by Mohammed (570-632). He was responsible for the dictum that where God created a disease, there he also created its cure; intemperance is the cause of all maladies with proper diet as the basis of all cures, and that anger causes illness.

With Muslim culture now centering in Damascus, one of its prime leaders was the Persian Geber Ibn Hajar (702-765), a keen innovator, who after developing a treatise on poisons derived from Dioscorides went on with metallurgical experiments with various alloys in order to try to get something like gold. This was the beginning of alchemy. By keeping the methods secret, the ersatz gold might be traded as real. The search for the philosopher's stone, by which base metals could be transmuted into gold, continued for many centuries. In his effort to dissolve metals and thus to control them, he developed what we call nitric acid and probably sulfuric acid (sour oil of vitriol), and their combination, aqua regia, which dissolves gold. By his technical descriptions of filtration, distillation, sublimation and the use of water baths, Geber may be said to have started chemistry.

Astrological ideas were important in all of this, with much esoteric symbolism so temptingly exciting, not only in later medieval times, but even in our own. Parts of the universal soul of the universe were supposed to dwell as spirits in everything. Some of these spirits could be driven out or extracted by fire or heat, as when quicksilver would run out of roasted cinnebar. One could obtain by heat the spirit of nitre, or by distillation, the spirit of wine. Indeed, the Arabic word *alcohol* means "finely divided spirit," so finely divided that as it comes from distilled wine, it is invisible until it condenses on cooling.

The seven days of the week having been arranged in respect to the sun, moon, and those other bodies in the heavens which change position (the planets we call Jupiter, Venus, Mercury, Mars and Saturn), it was then apparent that a similar hierarchy of the metals could be established in order of diminishing power of value, e.g. gold, silver, copper, tin, quicksilver, iron, and lead, in correspondence to the symbolism of the days of the week, and the moving bodies in the skies. The Muslim effort to transmute base metals into precious gold had one interesting result. Geber seems to have made a colloidal gold preparation, *aurum potible* as the medieval alchemists called it, or potable gold. As the analogy of value, this was thought to be a precious remedy for any serious disease. It is remarkable that it should recently be promoted as useful in arthritis.

In a similar way, the early Muslim alchemists thought that they could find a universal "elixir of life" to cure all disease and to promote longevity. This was a logical idea: wine was known to promote euphoria, to make sick people feel better, and to make oldsters pathetically feel young again. By distillation they extracted the spirit of wine, and found a concentrated essence or spirit, which, they noted, had these effects enhanced. It should be possible, they argued, further to refine this spirit in order to get the elixir of life. They were on the way to get rather pure ethyl alcohol. We now achieve this at much expense in such a product as vodka, when synthetically, by progressively hydrogenating and hydrating acetylene, we could produce it very inexpensively. Tax laws, however, interfere: synthetic ethanol is out since our tax laws have not yet caught up with our technology, as Carbon and Carbide Chemical Company discovered a few decades ago.

Geber was the earliest Arabic medical writer, his book on poisons, *Kitab as-sumum*, appeared about 750 AD. This exists in two manuscripts (Cairo Ms. Taymur, Tibb 393, and Ms. As'sd Efendi 2491, Halab), the first of which has been reproduced and translated into German by Alfred Siggel *(Das Buch der Gifte des Gaber ibn Hayyan,* Franz Steiner Verlag, Wiesbaden, 1958, 223 pp. and 193 double plates). Geber's intellectual ability is manifest in the skillful ordering of the text, and in the clarity with which he expounds the humoral pathology of the Graeco-Roman tradition, quoting Hippocrates, Aristotle and Galen. That he kept records of his patients is indicated by the case histories which he offers.

The first section of Geber's treatise describes the structure of the human body and the character and interrelations of the humors and temperaments when in disease they no longer function properly. He grades aliments as food-stuffs of the first order, spice and condiments of the second, drugs of the third, and poisons of the fourth. He classifies drugs and poisons into animal, vegetable and mineral categories, and describes thirty-eight animal, 266 vegetable and forty-five mineral agents, together with thirty-seven mixtures, spices and perfumes. Stating that drugs act by virtue of their qualities, Geber significantly and clearly indicates that the difference between a drug and a poison is a quantitative one, and that any drug can be poisonous if taken in large enough amounts. Siggel lists the various drugs described, with notations and identification. Many are similar to those recommended in the old Egyptian medical papyri, and most of them seem to have been taken chiefly from Dioscorides. New however, are bhang *(Cannabis sativa,* or maybe *Hyoscyamus niger), ergot (Secale cornutum)* and *ganz alqaiy,* equated with *strychnos nux vomica.* Among the mineral drugs are arsenic trioxide *(sakk),* borax *(tinkar),* quicksilver *(zibaq),* vitriol or copper or zinc sulfate *(zag),* and cinnebar, red mercuric sulfide *(zungufr).*

As Garrison points out, Geber's influence was long-lasting: even as late as the sixteenth century Paracelsus upheld Geber in believing that sulfur and salt are paramount in our bodies, and that as "the sun rules the heart, the moon the brain, Jupiter the liver, Saturn the spleen, Mercury the lungs, Mars the bile, Venus the kidneys," so the seven corresponding planetary metals and their compounds are curative specifically for diseases of those organs.

Muslim medical writers were characteristically methodical and systematic. They organized their vast accumulation of knowledge and ideas on drugs in effective and convenient ways. The brilliant Arabic scholar, Martin Levy, indicates how the Muslim physicians developed special literary forms for the systematization of their knowledge: 1) synonymic lists of materia medica in alphabetical order, a useful procedure when so many different names were associated with the same drug; 2) books on poisons and drug effects; 3) prescription formularies; 4) alphabetical lists of materia medica including methods of identification, tests for purity, and therapeutic uses, following the Dioscoridean tradition, and 5) tabulated synopses of drugs and their uses. They also furnished lists of drugs that might be substituted for each other if any were in short supply.

All of this indicates a high standard of skill on the part of pharmacists and physicians, with collated recording, and broad social culturation. The Muslim world was a civilized one in which the sick were well handled in clean and efficient hospitals, with nursing care, and well regulated drug service. Surgery, however, made little progress; the cautery was used instead of ligatures, and pus formation was thought to enhance healing.

Professor Levy has well translated and studied the Medical Formulary or Aqrāābādbīn of Al-Kindi (Madison, University of Wisconsin, 1966, 410 pp.) Aber Yūsuf Ya 'qūb ibn Ishāq Al-Kindī (800-870) came from Kufa, now in Iraq. After study at Baghdad, he became an outstanding philosophical teacher of the rationalistic Mu'tazilite sect. His voluminous writings include twenty-four medical treatises and some thirty-six on technology, including alchemy. Al-Kindī's *Kitāb fī-kīmīyā,* "Book on Chemistry," a treatise on distillation and perfumes, was translated into German by Karl Garbers (Leipzig, 1948). This contains 107 recipes for ointments, aromatic oils and perfumes, and for substitute preparations for expensive drugs.

Professor Levy's attention was directed to a hitherto unknown unique manuscript of Al-Kindī (3603, Aya Sofya Kutubkhame), a medical formulary or Aqrāābādbīn, containing 165 prescriptions. Professor Levy has given extensive commentary on each of the drugs, running alphabetically in Arabic from ijjās (plum, *Prunus armeniaca*) to yanbūt (bean trefoil, *Anagyris foetida*). A typical prescription (No. 158) using metallic ingredients for an eye salve reads:

> Collyrium of abn Muhammed for preserving the eyes. It strengthens and protects them.
> Tutty (impure zinc oxide) pounded and washed seven times with clear water and then put in a mortar –3 mithals (about 14 gm.)
> Antimony sulfide   1 mithqàl
> Iron pyrite   1 mithqàl
> It is soaked in water then pulverized, soaked in marojam juice and filtered over a fire. Sukk (a confection of dates, clove, cardamon and sandalwood) and one mithquàl is added to it. Then it is pulverized until dry. Use it then as a collyrium. It is helpful, with God's aid.

Eye salves of this kind with mineral ingredients remained popular into our own century.

The formulary of Al-Kindī indicates the meticulous care expected by Muslim physicians in the preparation of medicaments by pharmacists. This kind of care was already apparent in the old Egyptian formularies but seems to have been somewhat neglected in Greco-Roman times. As Professor Levy suggests, the Muslim Aqrāābādbīn, or formulary, may have had its organizational inspiration from Galen's *De compositione medicamentorum,* as it was known in medieval Europe. Yet, the form and arrangement of the prescriptions was established long before this in the Egyptian Ebers, Hearst, London and Berlin medical papyri, as well as in the Babylonian medical clay tablets. There may well have been a long tradition of such prescriptions transmitted orally or in family records.

There remain many other Muslim formularies of drugs arranged in the conventional style so well established by Al-Kindī and his pharmacist contemporaries. Even the great Persian clinician of Baghdad, Al-Razi (860-932), compiled one. The ninth book of his huge *El Hacoi* (which was translated in 1297 into Latin and published in 1846) is devoted to drug therapy. This was influential even in the Renaissance. The Muslim formulary style was adapted in Latin by Pietro Abano (1250-1316) and remained popular for centuries.

As Professor Levy indicates, the Muslim lists of synonyms for drugs is of great importance in identification, the names being given in Greek, Hindi, Berber and other languages related to the origins of the drugs. A well known list of this sort was made by Moses Maimonides (1135-1204), the great hygienic teacher of Cordoba in the Western Caliphate. This lists 408 drugs with much detail on their sources and names. Significantly, this was entitled "Explanation of the Names of Drugs."

Levy emphasizes (*Bull Hist Med, 37*:130-138, 1963) the importance of the linguistic skill of Muslim medical writers in the identification of drugs used by the multitude of differing linguistic peoples in their culture. He illustrates fully with discussions on anise, *Pimpirella anisum;* castor bean plant, *Ricinus communis;* the pomegranate, *Punica gramatum,* and mustard, *Sinapis alba.* About a third of Al-Kindī's drugs come from Mesopotamia, 23 percent from Greek sources, 18 percent from Persia, 13 percent from India and 3 percent from ancient Egypt. There must be much overlap: My own knowledge of the drugs used by the old Egyptians suggests that about half or more of the plant, animal and mineral materials used by Muslim physicians and prepared by their pharmacists are to be found in the old Egyptian medical papyri.

The climax of Muslim drug compendia came with the appearance in 1260 of the Minhāj al-Dukkan of the Jewish Cairo pharmacist, Abū al-Muna ibn al-Attār. This remained standard into our own times in Arabic countries. It has been analyzed and described by Sami Hamarneh (*Bull Hist Med, 42*:450-461, 1968). Ostensibly writing to his son, al-Attār's drug manual became widely used and appreciated. Combining wise advice on educational effort, social obligations and professional deportment with clear practical information on drugs and their use, its long success was well justified.

The bulk of Al-Attār's treatise is devoted to collecting, identifying, preparing, preserving and using plant, animal and mineral drugs. Dosage forms are described, as well as the weights and measures used. Various tests are given to detect fraud or adulteration. Since many important drugs might be difficult to obtain, information is offered regarding substitutes that may be used.

Diet and the principles of drug therapy are discussed, as well as details of the properties of each drug arranged alphabetically. The value of Al-Attār's effort is clear from Hamarneh's statement that "This manuel continued from the late thirteenth through the nineteenth centuries to be one of the texts most consulted by apothecaries of Egypt and neighboring countries."

All the great Muslim physicians wrote on drugs. In the Baghdad Caliphate, Rhazes (860-932), the great Persian clinician who described smallpox so well (and by implication differentiated it from large pox) wrote a treatise on drug substitution. The Zoroastrian Haly Ben Abbas (d. 994) gave a synopsis of drugs and their uses in his *Almaleki*. The greatest of these Persian Muslim physicians was Ibn Sina, or Avicenna (980-1037), a congenial and successful court physician, a poet, a geologist, and a systematic classifier of the medical knowledge of his time. His *Canon*, a huge treatise, was very popular in medieval Europe and even in the Renaissance, going into sixteen Latin editions from 1473 to 1608 with the growth of printing. He recommended wine for wound dressing. The fifth book of the *Canon* describes in meticulous classified detail the medicaments in common use, their composition, indications for therapy, dosage, administration and toxicity. This follows the Aqrāābādbīn style of contemporary pharmacy treatises. It seems that the Muslim hospital pharmacies were under medical supervision, but that this did not apply to the public drug stores in the cities.

The physicians of the Western Caliphate, centering in Cordoba, contributed little original knowledge of drugs. Avenzoar (d. 1162) questioned Galenical dogmatism, was a keen clinician and recommended milk in phthisis. The wise hygienist, Moses Maimonides (1135-1204), wrote a tract on poisons and venoms, promoted balanced diets and introduced rhubarb as a mild laxative. He also compiled an explanation of the names of drugs.

A drug formulary under the authorship of a mysterious Mesue was compiled in Latin in the eleventh century and became very popular in medieval Europe. There seems to be no Arabic original. The Gondisapor tradition appears to be embodied in Mesue, his alleged son Ibn Sarabioun (Serapion) and in Honien ibn Ishaq (309-877), known to medieval Europe as Johannitius. All of these seem to have prepared formularies and drug lists which for some unknown reasons were early translated into Latin and became widespread in medieval Europe. Maybe the Nestorians at Gondisapor held an alluring fascination for the often freethinking physicians of medieval Europe.

The Mesue formulary classifies purgative drugs into mild (aloes, rhubarb, senna and wormwood), laxative (cassia, figs, prunes, tamarinds) and drastic (castor oil, colocynth, jalap, scammony). This was first printed in Venice in 1471 and went to more than thirty editions by 1581. Clearly it was influential.

The eminent toxicologist, Eduard Rudolf Kobert (1854-1918), stimulated many of his students at Dorpat to undertake historical studies. One was Abdul-Chalig Achimdow of Baku who translated an Arabic manuscript of Abu Mansur dated 1055 (*Historische Studien aus dem Pharmakologischen Institute der Kaiserlichen Universitat Dorpat,* Vol. III, pp. 137-414, 1893, with comments by Paul Horn and J. Jolly, with a bibliography of fifty items). This contains full descriptions of 584 drugs, 466 plants, forty-four animals and seventy-four minerals. The most extensive Muslim materia medica was the *Jami,* compiled by Ibn Baitar in the thirteenth century and listing about 1400 drugs.

The great medical historian, Moritz Steinschneider (1817-1907) made many contributions to our knowledge of Muslim medicine, published in *Virchow's Archiv fur Pathologische Anatomie* and elsewhere from 1871 to 1900. He traced particularly the continuing influence of the Dioscoridean tradition through Gondisapor to the famed hospital teaching centers at Baghdad, Cairo and Cordoba. Lucien LeClerc (1816-1893) had first emphasized this continuity (*Historie de la médicine Arabe,* Paris, 1876). He concludes that Dioscorides was a dominating influence. Another excellent discussion of *Arabic Medicine* (Cambridge University Press, 1921) was given by the eminent orientalist, Eward Granville Browne (1862-1926).

Already by the tenth century there was much specialization in the Muslim health professions. Pharmacy was independent. Professional regulations, as well as standards of measurement were enforced, usually by the high principles of the druggists themselves. Surgeons, ophthalmologists and veterinarians were also independent. Alchemy was also separate from medicine and pharmacy. Yet, pharmacists, by virtue of their skill in obtaining, classifying and preparing drugs, served all.

It is clear that there continued to be a continual flow of information on drugs from China, India, Mesopotamia and Egypt, through the Greco-Roman writers, particularly Dioscorides and Galen, into the Byzantine and Muslim eras. The decay of Rome did not stop the intellectual health effort. The Muslims classified, codified and added to the vast store of knowledge on drugs which had accumulated and had it ready to flow back into Europe again.

CHAPTER 6

DRUGS IN MEDIEVAL EUROPE

> Not poppy nor mandragora,
> Nor all the drowsy syrups of the world,
> Shall ever medicine thee to that sweet sleep
> Which thou hadst yesterday.
>
> WILLIAM SHAKESPEARE (1564-1616)
> *Othello*, III, iii.

In the Middle Ages, there was true "consent of the governed. Even before the downfall of the Western Roman Empire, Greek science was practically dead . . . Europe (was) practically nationless, at the mercy of wandering barbarians, her peoples terrae filii, adscripts of the glebe, "the different children of the earth" . . . The social history of Europe for several centuries was the up building of organized nations from loose tribal groups. In the welter of race immixture and race-absorption which ensued, the greatest need of European humanity was for a spiritual uplift, for regeneration and renewal of character rather than for intellectual development . . . Thus, the Christian Church with its spiritual appeal, its attractive symbolism, its splendid organization, and its consolidation with Feudalism in protecting Europe from Moslem invasion, could not but triumph."

FIELDING GARRISON

THE MIDDLE AGES OF EUROPE go roughly from the tenth to the fifteenth centuries of our era—a time of authoritarianism and feudalism, of heresis and chivalry, when hospitals and nursing grew from monasteries and convents, when plant drugs were gathered in the fields and sometimes grown in gardens, and when new technologies developed for preparing and preserving drugs for administration by mouth or by application to the skin. While most of this was extension of Graeco-Roman and Muslim knowledge, it was greatly aided by trade and by many teaching compendia.

The situation regarding drugs in medieval Europe can only be appreciated by some realization of the intellectual complexity of the period. The old well-established Roman peace and security were gone; epidemics, squalor, poverty and ignorance were everywhere. All thought focused on faith in the emotional teaching of salvation through the Church; the health professions almost vanished, and drug use returned to a primitive empiricism.

Many new folklore remedies were introduced through the Germanic tribes. Some of these folk-remedies were described by W. Demitsch and A.A. Henrici *(Hist Stud Pharmakol Inst Dorpat,* I, 1889 and IV, 1894). Mead supplanted wines and beers as the favored beverage. Hallucinating and poisonous mushrooms were known. Chronic ergotism (St. Anthony's Fire) was almost endemic, as a result of eating breads made from smutty rye. Smallpox was rampant, and plague devastated the crowded, dirty towns where rats abounded.

What learning existed in medieval Europe centered in the cathedrals and monasteries where a semblance of culture was maintained by laborious hand copying of available manuscripts. Some of these were medical, and usually of practical interest in regard to drugs. Monasteries even began to develop drug gardens to assure a supply of plant remedies.

The conventional Graeco-Roman drug tradition, well organized by Muslim genius, came back into Europe chiefly through Salerno. This was an important trade center on the southwest coast of Italy. Here came traders from all over the known world. Probably as early as the ninth century, a hospital must have been established to care for those who became sick. Significantly this was not under Church control. Those who cared for the sick may have asked for reference works to help in their effort. Some of them may have taken apprentices to aid in the gradually increasing load. Thus, slowly a school of medicine grew. It remained independent of Church regulation.

The translating of various medical and drug compendia from Greek and Arabic into Latin, so that the hospital staff at Salerno could use them, began with Constantinus Africanus (1015-1087). Born in Carthage, and having travelled in Ethiopia, he may have been a Negro. He must have known Greek as well as Arabic since his Latin translations include the Hippocratic aphorisms, prognostics and regimen in acute diseases, as well as a practical compendium of Galen. From the Arabic he translated some ten large and small compendia, one of which was on technics of drug preparation. Others dealt with eye diseases, melancholia, coitus, elephantiasis and the stomach. That he was original in a practical way is indicated by his own books on the urine, fever, general and special diets and the properties of simple medicaments. The latter is a compendium of conventional Graeco-Roman and Muslim plant, animal and mineral drugs. A careful analysis of the writings of Constantine is given by H. Schipperges in his study of the assimilation of Arabic medicine into the Latin Middle Ages (*Sudhoffs Arch Gesch Med,* Beiheft 3, Steiner, Wiesbaden, 1964, 240 pp.). Constantine's work was influential and stimulated much effort at translating into Latin some of the Graeco-Roman classics which came in manuscript from the Crusades at a later time. This may have been a factor in the gradual rise of universities as at Paris (1110), Bologna (1113), Oxford (1167) and Montpelier (1181).

The Salerno Medical School prospered, however informally it may have started and developed. The hospital must have sheltered a great variety of diseased persons from the ships which came to trade. This must have given an excellent opportunity for clinical teaching without reliance on authority. Freedom from Church regulation promoted independent effort. The care of the sick was systematized and they were sent away with practical advice on how to keep well (Regimen Sanitatis). The school became coeducational. Anatomical study began as a background for surgery. Drug use was widely extended and organized.

The major writing on drugs from Salerno was the *Antidotarium* of Nicholas, who was active in the twelfth century. This was a formulary of 139 conventional prescriptions, often similar to those found in ancient Egyptian medical papyri. It included a table of weights and measures which established the apothecaries' system. Its contemporary popularity is indicated by the promptness with which it was so well printed (Venice, N. Jensen, 1471) when the presses came into use.

At about the same time appeared the *De simplici medicina* of Mathaeus Platearius, based on Dioscorides. This work inspired later French herbals. Another twelfth century drug compendium was the *Macer Floridus* of unknown authorship. This was a poem describing the virtues of some eighty-eight plant remedies. It was early printed as *De naturis qualitatibus et virtutibus octuaginta octo herbarum Neapoli*. The *Antidotarium* of Nicholas is usually quoted as the source (fol. 32 verse) of the famed *spongia sommifera*, the widely used anesthetic in medieval Europe. As Garrison so neatly summarizes, the soporific sponge was certainly pre-Salernitan; it occurs in the Mss. Bamberg *Antidotarium* of the ninth century, and in other manuscripts of about the same time. It may have developed from Dioscorides, and was noted by Avicenna, Isadore of Seville, and Jerome of Brunswick. The recipe calls for a sponge to be steeped in a water or wine mixture of opium, lettuce, hemlock, hyoscyamus, mulberry juice, mandragora and ivy. This was dried for storage and moistened when ready to be inhaled or its juice to be swallowed by the patient before operation. Sometimes belladonna or perhaps hemp was used instead of mandragora.

Salernitan surgery seems to have been practical and successful. Roger of Palermo (twelfth century) wrote a *Practica* about 1170 which became a text at Salerno. In it he prescribed ashes of sponges and seaweed (containing iodine) for goiter and used mercurial ointments for skin sores and lice. Teodorico Borgognoni (1205-1296) was Bishop of Cervia and distinguished himself by his sound surgical teaching. In opposition to conventional methods, he advocated cleanliness in wounds to reduce pus, using wine and distilled alcoholic preparations in dressing. He also used mercurial ointments for skin sores and recommended the *spongia sommifera* for anesthesia, as did the critical but pus-loving Guy de Chauliac (1300-1370). Indeed, the anesthetic sponge was well enough known that there are references to it in the contemporary literature from Boccaccio to Marlowe and Shakespeare.

After the success of the School of Salerno, many Church supported medical training programs were initiated. Toledo became a center for translating works directly from Arabic into Latin. The medical school at Montpelier flourished. Here practiced and taught Arnold of Villanova (1235-1311) who developed tinctures as effective ways of stabilizing crude drug preparations for administrations. He enthused over the health-giving properties of wines. He was among the first Europeans to develop distillations and to use herb distillates (cordials or liqueurs) as medicine. The monks became proficient in such preparations, some, as Chartreuse or Benedictine, persisting to this day.

In medieval Europe there was much effort locally to exploit indigenous drug lore. This occurred from England to Russia. English and Irish Leech-Books of herb medicine were compiled as early as the tenth century. Often they gave a pretense at authority by using copies of plant drugs derived from Italy, and descriptions from Pliny. Henrik Harpenstreng (d. 1244) compiled *Danske Laegebog* describing herb remedies, and a treatise on purgatives. The Aristotlean, Albertus Magnus (1143-1280) of Germany, wrote on plant remedies and inspired a work on cosmetics *(De secretis mulierum)*.

Recently, Alfred Von Henria of Helsingfors made a careful analysis of Russian folk-medicine, to which J. Alksnis added an account of Lettish medical lore. These appear as Vol. IV of *Historische Institute der Kaiserlichen Universität Dorpat,* (Halle, Tausch and Grosso, 1894, 295 pp.). This contains data on seventy-four plants used medically for various purposes, from various species of anthemis to verbascum, including gentian and spiraea. Some twenty folk remedies from animal sources are described, as well as ten from minerals. Most of this is similar to the folk-medicine developed and later codified in the eastern Mediteranean. Russian medicine in general developed from Byzantine sources.

Knowledge of drugs was widespread in medieval Europe, with much derived from local plant lore, and much from conventional Graeco-Roman and Muslim backgrounds. The drug trade must have been large. Monasteries developed herb gardens to counteract the efforts of drug mongers. They later became physic gardens to aid in identification of medicinal herbs. Venice developed a lucrative drug trade which later passed to Lisbon and London as explorations opened new ways to eastern drug sources.

Medieval Europe greatly expanded the extensive trade and public sale of drugs which so characterized Muslim medicine. With small bulk and easy preservation, the profits could be great. There was also much possibility for gain by taking advantage of general ignorance of the identity of drugs and of methods of adulterating them. There was much demand for drug compendia, and it is to the credit of medieval physicians that they tried earnestly to fill this need. Thus, the way was made ready for the standardization of drugs which came with the burgeoning intellectual awakening of the Renaissance.

CHAPTER 7

DRUG DEVELOPMENT IN THE RENAISSANCE

> Throw out opium . . .; throw out a few specifics . . .; throw out wine, which is a food, and the vapors which produce the miracle of anesthesia, and I firmly believe that if the whole materia medica, *as now used,* could be sunk to the bottom of the bottom of the sea, it would be all the better for mankind,—and all the worse for the fishes.
>
> OLIVER WENDELL HOLMES (1809-1894)
> *Medical Essays*

PERHAPS THE MOST CHARACTERISTIC factor in the intellectual flowering of the Renaissance was the development of printing. Spurred by the rising flood of eager young scholars demanding books for study, the manuscript copyists were swamped. Johann Gutenberg (1379-1468) and Johann Fust (1400-1466) developed printing from moveable type about 1454 in Mainz and issued the magnificent *Gutenberg Bible* about 1456. Following the sack of Mainz by the French, the early printers scattered. Printing was soon flourishing in Italy and France as well as in Germany, and books became relatively easy for students to acquire. The knowledge explosion was on the way.

Books printed before 1501 are arbitrarily but especially prized. Called *incunabula* or cradle-books, they were usually beautifully printed and often large (folio) in size. Among the incunabulae were many medical books, drug compendia and herbals. The latter were especially influential in exciting interest in plant drugs, their sources, identification, preparation and use.

An early printed herbal, illustrated though crudely, was the *Herbarius Moguntinus* printed by Peter Schoffer (1425-1502) in

Mainz in 1484. A year later Schoffer issued *Hortus sanitatis,* a compilation edited by a Johann von Kaub and put into German vernacular as *Gart der Gesundheit.* It included some five hundred very crude conventional plant pictures, but that was enough to stimulate wide interest which inevitably led to direct study of plants and their possible use as drugs. The *Hortus sanitatis* was translated into French as *Le grand herbier* and was the basis for later English herbals.

Actually the first printed herbal seems to have been *Herbarius Apuleius Platonicus,* a medieval compilation printed from a possible Salernitan manuscript at Monte Cassino, in 1480 by Filippo de Lignamine in Rome. Arnold Klebs (1870-1943) in his usual careful manner, prepared a *Catalogue of Early Herbals* (Lugarno, 1925).

Another factor which greatly stimulated interest in plant remedies, especially of a novel sort, were the great Reniassance exploratory voyagers. Repeatedly these returned to Europe with remarkable accounts of valuable new drugs from exotic places. The drug and spice trade became highly competitive. There was an ever growing demand for ready reference books for the identification and use of drugs. One of the first to be printed was the *Artzneibuch* by Ortolff of Wurzburg, written around 1400 but published by Zainer, probably in Augsburg in 1477. This pioneering drug manual was popular, as it was in the vernacular. Herbals came along rapidly and with continuing improvement of information and illustration.

The first to describe medicinal plants of the New World was F. de Oviedo, Viceroy of Mexico (1478-1557), who published his *Summaria* in Toledo in 1525. This was followed by the more complete discussion of Nicholas Monardes (1493-1588) in his *Dos Libros* issued in Sevilla in 1565. Meanwhile, Garcia de Huerta (1490-1570) published in Goa in 1563 his *Cologuios dos simples,* the first effort by a European to describe the rich indigenous plant drugs of India. This rare volume contains a classical account of cholera. An illustrated revision was issued by Cristovao Acosta (1515-1594?) under the title *Tratado de las drogues y medicinas de las Indias Orientales* (Burgos, 1578).

English herbals began with the anonymous ". . . *ye vertues & propyrtes of herbs,*" published by Rycharde Bankes in London in 1525. The first illustrated English herbal was *The grete herbal,* published by Travaris in Southwarke in 1526. A considerable scholar was the wine-loving and churchly contentious physician William Turner (1510-1568), who introduced a number of European drugs into English use in his *Libellus de re herbaria nova* (London, 1538). His *A Book of the Natures of All Wines* (New York City, Scholars Facsimilies, 1941) emphasized the health aspects of wines and cautioned against their abuse. As Sanford Larkey (1898-1969) indicates in his introduction to the reprint of Turner's treatise in wines, white wines were favored medicinally. To this book on wine, Turner added an account of the "great Treacle made by Andromachus; and of the Treacle Salt." This was taken from Galen, who was quoted at length. The Treacle Salt was for skin application and was made of various herbs mixed with salt. Turner did not list the many ingredients, and advised that apothecaries be consulted about it. Later, with extensive illustrations, Turner issued *A New Herbal,* in three volumes, published in London from 1551 to 1568. The last of these was dedicated to Queen Elizabeth, with whom Turner had once conversed in Latin! Turner's *Herbal* was one of the important scientific contributions of sixteenth century England. Another was his *Avium praecipuarur* (Cologne, 1544), a pioneering scientific ornithological treatise.

Another great English herbalist was John Gerarde (1545-1612) whose *Herbal or generall historie of plantes* was first published in London in 1597 and revised with corrections for publication in London in 1633. This described some 2800 plants, but seems to have been based on the *Cruydebosk* of Rembert Dodoens (1517-1585), first issued with illustrations in Antwerp in 1554. Dodoens also published a treatise on purgatives (Antwerp) and brought all his studies together in his *Stirpium historiae* (Antwerp, 1583). This was a huge volume with 1340 illustrations. He also gave a clear account of ergotism. The last of the English herbalists was the pun-loving John Parkinson (1567-1650) whose *Theatrum botanicum* appeared in London in 1840. This was a huge volume of 1755 pages and described 3,800 plants. The herbals were dying of their own weight.

The German herbalists are often called the fathers of botany. Their greatness was paced by Otto Brunfels (1488-1534) who followed Luther, and then, at age 65 received an M.D. degree from Basel and was appointed city physician in Berne. The illustrations to his three-volume *Herbarium vivae eicones* (Strassburg, 1530-40) were direct from nature, as were his own descriptions and comments. He thus was the first to discard the time-worn accounts and stereotyped illustrations coming from Graeco-Roman antiquity. Not quite as satisfactory from the standpoint of illustrations was the *Neue Kreuter Buch* (Strassburg, 1539) of Jerome Bock, called Tragus (1498-1554). Accurate and well illustrated, even for American plant drugs, was the famed *De historia stirpium commentarii* (Basel, 1542) of Leonhart Fuchs (1501-1566). He described the fox-glove, and fuchsias are named for him. The great humanistic bibliographer Conrad Gesner (1516-1565) prepared a pocket dictionary of plant drugs, *Historiae plantarum* (Paris, 1541), and a useful compendium of purgative agents, *Enumeratio medicamentorum purgantium* (Basel, 1543).

Gesner is especially to be remembered for his generous editing of the posthumous works of that brilliant Rhineland youth, Valerius Cordus (1514-1544), who had been so well trained by his physician father, Euricius (1486-1535). The latter had written a dialogue, *Botanologicon* (Cologne, 1534), in which he condemns pharmacists for falsely labelling drug receptacles with Greek names no longer applicable. He was also the author of the sharp quatrain *Tres facies habet medicus* which so well expresses the feelings of people toward members of the health professions:

> Three faces has the doctor;
> A god's when first he's sought
> And then an angel's, the cure half-wrought;
> But when comes due the doctor's fee,
> Then Satan looks less terrible than he!

Valerius Cordus had carefully edited Dioscorides and had added some five hundred new plant remedies, as a result of his extensive travels. Gesner issued this under the title, *Annotationes in Pedacii*

Dioscorides Anazarbei de materia medica (Strassburg, 1561).

This book contained a most important contribution from Cordus, *De artificiosis extractionibus,* which, in its freedom from magic and wishful thinking, and in the clear exposition of the techniques employed, marked the transition from the teleological efforts of alchemy to the rational empiricism of chemistry. This correctly described the preparation and properties of *oleum dulce vitrioli,* sweet oil of vitriol, which we call ether. This was obtained by distilling "strong biting wine" (alcohol) with "sour oil of vitriol" (sulfuric acid). Cordus carefully specified the character of the materials to be used, the apparatus, and the procedure to be followed. This was a far leap from the conventional secrecy and esoteric rites of the alchemists. Thinking the product to be a liquid sulfur, he noted its lack of color, its rapid evaporation, its tendency to cause, salivation, and its safety. He recommended it for the relief of cough and pneumonia.

Cordus is significant in any history of drug use for another achievement of his few years. He compiled the best *officially recognized* book of drug preparations, a *pharmacopeia.* True, a formulary, *Nuovo Receptario* (Firenze, 1498), written by Florentine physicians and apothecaries had been authorized as a reference book for their use, but it did not acquire anything comparable to the wide use of *Dispensatorium pharmacopolarum* of Valerius Cordus (Nuremberg, 1546). The Senate of the City of Nuremberg had requested this work, and on examining it, the publication of it was authorized, and apothecaries were ordered to make their preparations in accordance with its directions. It went into thirty-five editions and five translations. Soon it was followed by many other city pharmacopeias, including the famed Pharmacopeia Londinensis issued by the Royal College of Physicians in 1618. The first French pharmacopeia was the *Codex medicamentarius seu pharmacopeia Parisiensis* (Paris, 1639).

The first official American pharmacopeia was prepared by a small committee representing the various health professions under the active direction of Lyman Spaulding (1744-1821), a protege of the keen biomedical scientist Samuel Latham Mitchell (1764-1831). The latter had already prepared the New York Hospital

Pharmacopeia in 1815. A William Brown (1752-1792) had issued a systematic materia medica earlier *(Pharmacopeia simpliciorum et efficaciorum,* Philadelphia, 1788), but this had no organizational or official recognition. The American pharmacopeias were similar to their European predecessors in selecting for inclusion only those drugs and drug preparations considered by the committee to be useful. European pharmacopeias usually had two lists of drugs: the first (series medicaminum) being those which pharmacists were supposed always to have to be prepared on order. While gradually developing as reference sources for drug standards for purposes of identification and uniformity of product, the pharmacopeias were initially, and have since remained, alphabetized lists of drugs with some descriptive detail which are chosen by committees of experts on the basis of their collective judgment as to what drugs physicians should use in practice. Their official character depends on the fact that legal requirements permit governmental agencies to use only such items in the materia medica as are described in the respective pharmacopeias. This tends to inhibit the judgment of physicians in regard to prescribing drugs, especially new ones, which are not included in the pharmacopeia, or older drugs which for some reason (usually presumed lack of effectiveness) have been dropped. The net result has been a significant drop in the number of drugs and drug preparations in the pharmacopeias as the years have gone by, and in the number of drugs commonly used. It would seem, however, that there might wisely be for general reference use by members of the health professions, a set of accumulated agreed-upon standards for identification and purity of any and all drugs which have been or may be used medicinally. The closest to this is the *Merck Index,* the eighth edition of which (Rahway, 1968) contains over ten thousand items.

With so much Renaissance interest in plant drugs, it was quite natural that there should have been printed then many editions of Dioscorides. It is not always known from what manuscripts these were prepared, but most of them included copious commentaries by their Latin translators. As Garrison notes, the great illustrated Julia Anicia manuscript of the sixth century is in Vienna and has been reproduced. There is also an illustrated manuscript in the Morgan Library, New York City. There were Latin translations as early as the sixth century: a ninth century copy is in Munich, and another earlier one in Vienna. The latter was printed by Medenblich near Siena in 1478. The Greek text was printed by Aldus in Venice in 1499. A bilingual text was printed in Cologne in 1529.

It was Jean de la Ruelle (1474-1537) who made a popular Latin translation of Dioscorides, adding many new medicinal plants, with extensive commentary on the various names by which they were known (Paris, Stephanus, 1516). The most popular of the Latin commentators on Dioscorides was Pietro Mattioli (1501-1577) of Siena. He added some two hundred new medicinal plants, and used excellent wood-cut illustrations with detailed commentary. This appeared from the Guinta press (Venice, 1554) and went through many editions and translations, including Italian and Czech. The definitive text is by Max Wellman in three volumes (Berlin, 1906-1914).

An important feature of Renaissance intellectual curiosity was the beginning again of Aristotelian efforts at the classification of natural phenomena and objects. This could only be done as a result of their careful description. This was done for the heavens by the Polish physician Nicholas Copernicus (1473-1543) in his heliocentric classic, *De Revolutionibus orbium celestinum* (1543), which started modern astronomy. With the human body as the microcosm, this was accomplished in a grand manner by the Belgian Professor of Anatomy and Surgery at Padua, Andreas Vesalius (1514-1564) in his *Fabrica de corporis humain* (Basel, 1543). For the plant world, including medicinal herbs, this was begun by Andrea Cesalpino (1524-1603) of Pisa in his great *De Plantis* (Florence, 1583). In this he arranged about 1520 plants by their fruits into fifteen classes and distinguished between systematic and economic botany. The Italians claim him as the discoverer of blood circulation. He did propose the idea, but did nothing to develop or demonstrate it.

Vesalius is important in the history of pharmacology for his pioneering effort at drug standardization in order to assure some degree of uniformity in expected results from the use of any particular drug. This was an extension of the concept developed by Valerius Cordus in his pharmacopeia. The pharmacological work of Vesalius is to be found in *Epistola . . . radicis Chynae decocti* (Basel, 1546); it is a long-winded letter to his friend, Joachim Roelants (1496-1558), the printing of which (by Operinus of Basel, who printed the great Fabrica) was arranged by his brother, Franciscus. The letter describes the use of the China root by Vesalius in treating his royal patient, the great Hapsburg Emperor Charles V (1500-1558). This is well described in his customary meticulous manner by Charles D. O'Malley (1907-1970) in his brilliant biography *Andreas Vesalius of Brussels* (University of California, 1964).

The China root was introduced into Europe along with many other exotic remedies primarily for the purpose of treating what we usually call syphilis. This word was the fictional name of the hero of a poem, *Syphilis, sive Morbus Gallicus* (Venice, 1530) by the keen Veronese physician, Girolamo Fracastoro (1484-1553), who pioneered in the description of contagious disease. In the poem on the French disease, Fracastoro describes the symptoms of the disease in the hero of the poem so well that it went through many editions and resulted in the name of the hero of the poem becoming the name of the disease.

Syphilis is significant in the history of Renaissance drug use. The disorder was noted in Italy around 1493, just after the return of Columbus and his sailors from the second voyage to the New World. The disease spread rapidly. It was popularly thought to have come from the New World. Fracastoro discussed its etiology in his poem, and suggested that it may have been around for a long time, gradually losing virulence, until something triggered its contagiousness. He dismissed the contemporary astrological explanations as nonsense, but admitted the possibility of a New World origin. It has recently been proposed that yaws, endemic in the Caribbean area, and caused by a related treponema microorganism, though not venereal, may indeed have been brought home by the early voyagers, and this organism enhanced the virulence of the syphilitic one.

It is remarkable that as soon as the new French disease was recognized and described, the most effective remedy against it, mercurial ointment, was promptly recommended. This had been introduced by the tenth century by the Muslims for treatment of skin lesions, which may have included large pox.

On the generalization that natural remedies are to be found where peculiar diseases exist, New World plant drugs were brought to Europe to treat syphilis. Among these was guaiacum, the heart wood of *Guaiacum officinale,* a small resinous West Indian tree. This was made into a decoction, and became popular in treating syphilis in lieu of mercury ointment, which was likely to cause salivation, tooth loss, and other toxic symptoms. The great artist, Benvenuto Cellini (1500-1571) in his famed *Autobiography,* describes his experience with syphilis and its treatment. The active agent in guaiacum is a resin containing guaiaconic acid ($C_{20}H_{24}O_5$), which induces sweating and urination; these may have been useful in fevers. It has no spirochaeticidal action, as is the case with mercury ointment. It seems to have had merely palliative effect on syphilis, which is relatively self-limiting within a few weeks as far as the first and second stages are concerned.

Several substitutes for guaiacum appeared. These were various kinds of brown and wrinkled smilax roots, and also the chippy roots of sassafras. The chief smilax were the roots of *Smilax medica* from Mexico, *S. ornata* from Jamaica, and *S. officinalis* from Honduras. This was sarsaparilla. While sassafras is a small deciduous tree from Venezuela, the smilax are woody vines related to laurel. These three antisyphilitic drugs, smilax, sarsaparilla and sassafras were called, in the sixteenth century in Europe, "nature's own remedies" or "blood purifiers." They are still so-called in the proprietary preparation, S.S.S., sold over-the-counter in American drug stores.

From India, or maybe China, came a similar smilax root, the China root, *Radix chinae,* from *Smilax China* or *S. glabra*. It was of this that Vesalius wrote. He describes how he used it in treating some of his patients and discusses its properties at length in comparison with guaiacum and other similar crude woody roots from the New World. He notes correctly the irregular oval and flattened roots, wrinkled brown on the outside, and mealy whitish within with no odor or taste. He contrasts this with the root of spartaparilla, our sarsaparilla, a woody vine brought by merchants from Lusitania (Portugal). This would be the dried root of a smilax, of which there are some two hundred species. Vesalius correctly, but wordily, describes the differences between his specimen of sarsaparilla and China root.

The care used by Vesalius in describing China root and guaiacum and sarsaparilla indicates his interest in the accurate identification of drugs for satisfactory and consistent clinical effectiveness. This, with meticulous instructions he gives for their use, shows him to have been a pioneer in the development of rational drug use which is what pharmacology is all about. Vesalius is renowned as the founder of modern human anatomy. He deserves consideration also as a pioneer in a less elusive and more objectively oriented science, modern pharmacology.

Vesalius' great anatomical discoveries were promptly applied in surgery, especially by the keen and sympathetic surgeon, Ambrose Paré (1510-1590). Paré was also interested in drugs. He described what must have been carbon monoxide poisoning, noting the bright red blood and skin. In his *Discours a savoir de la mennie* (Paris, 1582), he ridiculed the use of presumed magical remedies, such as powdered unicorn or mummy, showing the quackery involved.

The most influential person in regard to drugs during the Renaissance was that truculent Swiss, Auereolus Theophrastus Bombastus von Hohenheim (1493-1541) or Paracelsus, as he called himself. Son of a book-loving physician, Paracelsus earned his doctoral degree under the medical humanist, Leonicenus (1428-1524), at Ferrara in 1515. After much wandering, in which he learned popular medicine at first hand, he was appointed Professor of Medicine at Basel in 1527, and at once was in the midst of trouble and controversy. He is thought to have died from a wound received in a tavern brawl in Salzburg. His writings were extensive, often obscure, and widely respected.

One of the famed rough German statements of Paracelsus indicates appreciation of the dose-effect relation in drugs: "All things are poisonous, and nothing is without poisonous effect; the dose is what makes anything poisonous or not poisonous." Paracelsus introduced distilled oils of aromatic plants as remedies. He also popularized tinctures. It is unlikely that he developed laudanum, the tincture of opium, although he is reputed to have praised it. Paracelsus elaborated a fantastic theory of therapy on the basis of Geber's basic chemical agents of combustible sulfur, volatile mercury, and residual salt. There is discussion about Paracelsus possibly using the pseudonym of Basil Valentine to introduce into medical use such chemical agents as sugar of lead, (lead acetate), muriatic acid (hydrochloric acid), ammonia, sour oil of vitriol (sulfuric acid), and antimony salts. The *Currus triumphalis antimonii* (Basel, 1604) led to the wide use of antimony salts as emetics and diaphoretics at the start of fevers. Certainly mystical alchemy was gradually becoming empirical chemistry, and pure chemical compounds were beginning to replace the complex crude drug mixtures, such as theriacae of the ancients. Paracelsus deserves the credit for much of this transition.

Paracelsus thought that sulfur was a prime remedy. He apparently thought that the sweet oil of vitriol (ether), prepared by Valerius Cordus, was the essence of sulfur. He says *(Defensiones, in Four Treatises of Theophrastus von Hohenheim called Paracelsus,* by O. L. Temkin, G. Rosen, G. Zilboorg and H. E. Sigerist, Boston, Johns Hopkins Press, 1941), "But here this should be known of that sulfur: among them all the one from vitriol is the most notable, because it is fixed by itself; furthermore, this sulfur has such a sweet taste, that even chickens will take it, whereupon they sleep for a while and awaken without injury." Here then was experimental evidence for the anesthetic power of ether three centuries before its application in surgery. Paracelsus was a keen observer and a skilled physician and surgeon.

He noted the lung disorders of miners, ascribing the symptoms to continued exposure to the dusts in mines. He also had analyzed mineral baths and recommended their use in skin disorders. He used gallic acid or tannin to precipitate iron salts and suggested them in anemias. The *specificum purgans Paracelsi*, which he introduced, is potassium sulfate. He used alum as a styptic and differentiated it from astringent iron salts. He also recommended arsenical, mercurial and copper salts as astringents. Mercury he considered to be specifically curative of syphilis. Paracelsus may well be said to have begun the modern era of the use of pure chemical agents as drugs. He was a high point in protopharmacology.

An unpleasant aspect of Renaissance protopharmacology was the rise of homicidal poisoning. This occurred with the introduction of arsenic trioxide, commonly called arsenic. This white substance is readily water soluble and being without taste or odor can be taken in wine or beverage without detection. It is not known when this became popularly available. Certainly during the Renaissance there must have been confusion between intestinal infections and deliberate poisoning. Food poisoning and cholera must have been as prevalent then as now. The sudden onset of food poisoning and its distressing symptoms must easily have aroused suspicion of deliberate poisoning. But Renaissance rings have come down to us with hidden receptacles in which arsenic trioxide powder could be concealed.

Intriguing are the many tales of murder by poisoning, especially on the part of the Borgias, that powerful Italian family which manipulated Papacy and Empire. Even Leonardo da Vinci (1453-1519), that amazing artist and scientist, experimented with poisons. He knew the toxic power of arsenic trioxide. Wondering if it could be absorbed into plants or fruits from the ground or by injection into the trunk, he made the direct experiment of using a peach tree. He failed to find any toxicity in the peaches when fed to animals.

The most fascinating account of Leonardo is by Dimitri Merezhkowski (1865-1941) in the book entitled, in its excellent English translation by B. G. Guerney, *The Romance of Leonardo* (New York, Modern Library, 1928). Charles Singer (1876-1965), the great historian of science, once told me that Merezhkowski's *Leonardo* evokes the swirling emotional and intellectual confusion and clashes of the Renaissance more accurately than any other record. It clearly contrasts the popular superstitious faiths of the common people with the growing rationalism of the

Renaissance intellectuals. One of its most brilliant passages describes the Witches' Sabbath, with skin inunction of mixtures of belladonna, hemp, and other brain-disturbing drugs to result in the wild hallucinations of the Walpurgis Night, and the subsequent exhaustion and apathy.

It was not mere coincidence that Leonardo should have known about arsenic trioxide, or have become so interested in anatomy, or to have had so critical an opinion of medical practice; he was a member of the Guild of St. Luke, the craft guild for physicians and apothecaries. Graphic and plastic artists belonged to this guild also, since it was from the apothecaries that they obtained their pigments, oils, solvents, clays and other materials for their craft. Thus, in the Renaissance the health professions with their growing scientific background were closer to the art community than at any other time.

The intellectual vigor of the Renaissance, in spite of Reformation, Counter-Reformation, and disruptive religious warfare, carried into the seventeenth century. Indeed, the first half of the seventeenth century may be considered to have witnessed the transition to the Baroque culture of the late seventeenth and early eighteenth centuries, with the rise of nationalism and of powerful experimentation in every line of endeavor, including drugs.

CHAPTER 8

DRUGS IN THE SEVENTEENTH AND EIGHTEENTH CENTURIES

> One should treat as many patients as possible with a new drug while it still had the power to heal.
>
> WILLIAM OSLER (1849-1919)

THE GREAT BAROQUE CULTURE in Europe was one of consolidation, as in the nationalistic effort; of individual genius, as with Shakespeare, Cervantes, Rembrandt, Bach, Moliere, and Newton; of quantitation in science, as with Harvey, Galileo and Boyle; of trade and affluence, and of architectural grace. The drug trade boomed, and the Dutch wrested it from the Portugese making exponential profits from the East Indies. Economic pharmacology flourished, although with few available records. Cautious systematic experiments with drug effects began, and there was wide effort at standardization, at least for local drug use. Units of measurement varied greatly, and fortunes were made by shrewd traders who knew where to buy when supplies were long, and when to sell where they were short. The modern world was dawning, even though the economy remained agricultural and cities were just beginning to grow in spite of plagues and epidemics.

Characteristic of the period were new drugs from far away. The spices were widely used, not merely for flavoring, but for alleged health benefit also. Most of the spices do have digestive effect and they improve gastric and intestinal secretion and motility. It is interesting that the use of condiments and carminatives should have flourished so continuously from the time of the ancient Egyptian formularies. Their use was popularized, and grocers carried them as well as apothecaries. There was bound to be much adulteration and variation, so that some effort at standardization was demanded for popular as well as prescription use.

The Portugese tried to keep secret the trade-route to the Far East, but the Dutch found the way and possessed the sources. They monopolized the Banda Island trade in nutmeg and mace (from *Myristica fragrans*) and hoarded the entire crop in Amsterdam for years, selling at fantastic prices. They seized Molucca for its cloves *(Eugenia or Caryophyllus aromaticus)*. Planting the trees on Amboyna which they could guard more readily, they destroyed all on the Moluccas. Further, they succeeded in monopolizing the Ceylon trade in cinnamon *(Cinnamomum zeylainum)*. Only slowly did the English gain a foot-hold in the spice and drug trade of India after the organization of the East India Company in 1600.

Thanks to the blessed fine print in Garrison *(Intro Hist Med,* 4th ed., Philadelphia, 1929, p. 293), one may find reference to a series of tracts issued in London in the latter part of the seventeenth century by a John Pechey of Gloustershire *(Index Catalogue Surg Gen Off,* 1st series, X:594-595). These describe new crude drugs from many places, but the names reveal little of what they are. Ginseng, for example, may be the roots of the Chinese *Panax ginseng,* or its North American cousin, *Panax quinquefolium,* now cultivated in Wisconsin for export to China. In Chinese folk-medicine this is a cure-all; the more its forked and branched root resembles the human body, the more powerful it is supposed to be. It contains much starch and gum, some resin and volatile oil, and a yellow sweetish panaquilon ($C_{12} H_{25} O_9$), soluble in alcohol and precipitated by water. Chinese and Russian pharmacologists are now claiming ginseng has hypotensive and tranquilizing effects. Cassine was the name of the dried leaves of the North American Virginia coast tree, *Ilex cassine,* which contains tannin and about 0.5 percent caffeine. This was a widely used drink of Amerinds.

Blatta bizantina seems to have been dried cockroach; this oily preparation was used on warts, skin eruptions and boils. Pliny at the beginning of our era recommended this by mouth for dyspnoea, and late in the nineteenth century, it was used in Russia as a diuretic and to control albuminuria. Salep was the name commonly given to a starchy root from various species of *Orchis* found in Southern Asia. A mucilage made from it was used to allay stomach irritation. Colombo wood was probably cinnamon, as Molucea nuts were probably cloves, and Bengala beans may have come from the sacred Hindu Bael tree *(Aegle marmelos)* whose leaves and fruit contain enough tannin to make it useful in controlling diarrhea and dysentery. Malabar nuts must have been *Cardamomum malabaricum* from India, used as a stomachtic or carminative even in ancient Egypt. In addition to a camphoraceous volatile oil, it is unusual for containing manganese compounds.

Angola seed, Maldive nuts, Ceylonian plant, Perigua, and casumar root cannot be traced. Names, as well as sources, are important in drug identification, as Dioscorides had recognized many centuries before.

Two of the most important drugs introduced into Europe in the seventeenth century were ipecacuanha and cinchona bark. The former was first described by Wilhelm Piso (1611-1678) of Leyden in his *Historia naturalis Brasiliae* (Amsterdam, 1648). It was lauded by J. C. A. Helvetius (1685-1755) in his *Recuil des Methodus pour la Guerison de Diverses Maladies* (The Hague, 1710) as the best remedy for diarrhea and dysentery. A decoction of ipecac root was used. This was found to have emetic properties, and as it was relatively safe, it supplanted the potentially toxic antimony emetics. It contains the alkaloid, emetine, widely used by the British as a specifically curative agent in amoebic dysentery or amebic abscess. We showed, however, (*JAMA, 98:*195, Jan. 16, 1932) that the effective dose of emetine damages cardiac muscle, and we introduced more satisfactory chemotherapeutic agents for amebiasis.

The complicated story of the introduction of cinchona (Jesuits; Peruvian) bark—often merely The Bark—into Europe has been reviewed by B. Holmstedt and G. Liljestrand in *Readings in Pharmacology* (Oxford, 1963, pp. 41-50), and well told by M.L. Duran-Reynolds in her *The Fever Bark Tree; the Pageant of Quinine,* (New York, 1946). The early history of cinchona has been well analyzed by A. W. Haggis *(Bull Hist Med, 10:*417, 568, 1941). Confusion with Peruvian balsam *(Toluifera Pereirae),* itself confused with balsam of Tolu *(Toluifera balsamum)*, often made for difficulty in the seventeenth century in judging which was really helpful in treating fevers. Gradually it was recognized that it was The Bark that seemed to cure all fevers, regardless of presumed cause or theory. It was largely the influence of that great English empiricist physician, Thomas Sydenham (1624-1689), that resulted in the practical success of The Bark in treating fevers, regardless of the long doctrine of the four humors, and in overthrowing Galenical theory and its dominance.

Cinchona, ipecac, Balsam of Peru and other South American native drugs were slowly introduced into Europe because the Spanish conquerors allowed no visitors, and tried to monopolize South American trade. How The Bark was smuggled out of Peru is not known. Its secret was really not revealed until Louis XIV (1638-1714) bought it from an English quack, Robert Talbor (1642-1681). It was finally clarified by Nicholas de Blegny (1652-1722) in his *Le Remede Anglois pour la Guerison des Fievres* (Paris, 1682). Here Talbor's prescriptions were given, and the conclusion was drawn that quinquina, as The Bark was called, is a specific febrifuge. It was the Italian pharmacologist Francesco Torti (1658-1741) who showed its curative specificity in malaria.

The heavy demand for The Bark threatened to exhaust the Peruvian source, and during the nineteenth century many attempts were made to smuggle seeds or plants to other tropical areas. It was Clements Markham (1830-1916) who finally succeeded in 1860 against great odds. The British in India, however, were negligent, and the Dutch finally developed great cinchona plantations in Java. When the Japanese seized Java in World War II, supplies of cinchona were cut, necessitating the development of satisfactory substitutes, as will be discussed later. With malaria remaining the most wide-spread endemic disease, and with the recognition of the specific curative effect of cinchona in malaria, the economic importance of The Bark continued. The story of The Bark is a complex one, and it well illustrates the vicissitudes of drug knowledge from the empirical lore of a native people to the commercialized rationality of the sophisticated present.

The widely used common beverages, tea, coffee, and cocao, have similar histories. The longest known is tea, the dried leaves of *Thea sirrensis,* from China; then coffee, the dried ripe seed of *Coffea arabica* from northeast Africa or *Coffea liberica* from west coastal Africa, and the cacao, the dried ripe seeds of *Cacao sativa* or *C. theobroma,* from tropical America. All three were used from antiquity in watery decoctions as mild stimulants and diuretics. All three contain related active substances which have these effects.

Some species of *Ilex* have also been used indigenously for these purposes and contain similar active agents. An example is mate, or Paraguay tea, the dried leaves of *Ilex paraguensis.* Another is cassine, the dried leaves of *Ilex cassine,* a highly regarded medicinal agent among North American natives.

Coffee, tea and chocolate, or cacao, gradually became popular in Europe during the seventeenth and eighteenth centuries. They came with ever increasing trade. Coffee houses in London rivalled the taverns and public houses where only alcoholic beverages were served. The mild mental stimulation of coffee started the wits of the day well on their way. Tea became popular in the afternoon, as it still is, for the tannin in it is enough to allay appetite. Chocolate became a French and Italian delight. In coffee, tea, and cacao one may note an excellent example of how popular tastes may determine wide-spread use of materials containing potentially powerful drugs, quite as in the case of alcoholic beverages.

Other exotic tropical plant drugs were becoming known in Europe, if only by rumor. Arrow poisons from the Amazon area were called by various names, gradually settling on curare. Another arrow poison from East Africa came from the seeds of a woody vine and was known as strophanthus. From a West African woody climber came the feared ordeal bean, or Calabar bean, carried by slaves to the Americas for esoteric use in determining guilt; if one survived after ingesting it, one was innocent. From South America came another bean, Jaborandi or Pilocarpus, or Paraguay bean. These were all exotic curiosities until the nineteenth century, when technical methods were devised for studying their biological effects and for isolating from them the chemical substances responsible for their biological action.

A full report on native medicinal plants from Brazil was made by Bernardino Antonio Gomez (1768-1823). This has recently been reprinted with a helpful introductory note by Jose A. do Valle, Professor of Pharmacology at the University of Sao Paulo *(Plantas Medicinais do Brazil,* Sao Paulo, 1972). This contains a life of Gomez by Olympio da Fonseca, a reproduction of the Lisbon 1801 edition of Gomez' report on ipecacuanha, and of the well illustrated Rio de Janeiro 1809 account of the medicinal plants of Brazil.

One of the most important plant drugs, digitalis, was introduced into rational clinical use during the late eighteenth century by William Withering (1741-1799) of Birmingham, England. His important discovery was due to his skill as a botanist. Withering was one of that brilliant group of British empirical physicians influenced by their hard-driving observant friend, the great pathologist, John Hunter (1728-1793), who helped to start controlled clinical experimentation.

Withering had already shown scientific leadership in mineralogy and chemistry; a mineral, barium carbonate, is named Witherite for him, and he analyzed mineral waters. He compiled *A Botanical Arrangement of all The Vegetables Naturally Growing in Great Britain* (London, 2 Vols. 1776). As a clinician, his skill was evident in his account of scarlet fever and its contagiousness. He was puzzled by his failure to provide relief for dropsy. Some of his patients seemed to be miraculously cured after taking a decoction of a dried herb mixture supplied by one of the "wise old women" of the neighborhood. Obtaining the material, he laboriously separated the dried leaf fragments of the several ingredients and was able to identify them microscopically.

Withering then tried decoctions of each of the ingredients separately in his patients, and found the one that worked—the leaves of the purple fox-glove, *Digitalis purpurea*. His classic report was *An Account of the Foxglove and Some of its Medical Uses* (Birmingham, 1785). In it he describes his study and his clinical findings. His advice on how to give digitalis for dropsy is still pertinent in assaying the drug directly on the patient; give digitalis until there is an effect on the heart, on the kidneys, on the stomach or on the brain. These are in order of increasing dosage. Withering

Drugs in the Seventeenth and Eighteenth Centuries

realized from the well-known but still theoretical demonstration of blood circulation by William Harvey (1578-1657) that digitalis, by slowing the heart, improves circulation, and thus increases urinary outflow and relieves dropsy. The effects of digitalis on the stomach and brain result from near toxic doses.

However, as Withering noted, not all his dropsical patients improved with digitalis, even though their hearts slowed. The differentiation between cardiac dropsy and renal dropsy was later made by Richard Bright (1789-1858), who demonstrated the pathological character of the latter. Bright's clinical study later led to the discovery of renin and angiotensin, and other active polypeptides.

It is interesting that in spite of all our detailed scientific effort to develop pure chemical digitaloids for precise clinical use, we still find the crude extract, dried powdered leaves, or the tincture of digitalis satisfactory for therapy in cardiac insufficiencies. Withering's study remains a landmark in the history of pharmacology as a prime example of the sound empirical use of a crude drug. His criteria for its administration are still valid.

Among the friends of John Hunter and William Withering was Thomas Percival (1740-1804) of Manchester. It was he who developed the codified rules for decent behavior between the members of the health professions, which he misnamed Medical Ethics. A sympathetic physician, he tried to ameliorate malnutrition among the exploited millworkers who were the grist of the Industrial Revolution. He introduced cod-liver oil as a supplementary nutrient, with no prescience of its future significance in pharmacology.

Another of this circle of friends, all within Edinburgh and London associations, was Edward Jenner (1749-1823) of Gloucestershire. He was a sharp observer of endemic smallpox and noted that milkmaids never got the disease. However, he found that they usually acquired a slight skin eruption, cowpox, soon after beginning to milk, and that the udders of cows often showed pustules, suggesting the source of contagion. The idea of skin inoculation of healthy people with pus from smallpox sores had long been considered, such as in writings from Salerno. Such inoculations had been practiced in England and Massachusetts in the early eighteenth century. Jenner used cowpox for inoculation on James Phipps in 1796, and and then made the real test with smallpox. The cowpox protected against the smallpox. In 1798, Jenner published twenty-three case reports, all successful, in his *Inquiry into the Causes and Effects of the Variolae Vaccinae* (London, 1798). In this, Jenner noted what we now call anaphylaxis.

As Garrison says, "Jenner transformed a local country tradition into a viable prophylactic principle." His report promptly stimulated wide use of cowpox inoculation against smallpox, and laid the basis for the concepts of preventive medicine and of public health. It also laid a foundation for the study of immunology, coming now in pharmacology to a consideration of the chemical characteristics and action of the immune bodies, which Jenner suggested are due to a permanent change in the blood following inoculation. Currently there is great pharmacological effort directed toward the control of immune processes by drugs.

Actually it was William Harvey (1578-1657) who successfully demonstrated the scientific methodology which began to flower during the late seventeenth and in the eighteenth centuries. A testy Englishman, trained at Padua, Harvey spent over a dozen years carefully experimenting with all kinds of animals, invertebrate and vertebrate, before reaching his conclusion that the blood in our bodies circulates by means of the pumping activity of our hearts. His *Excercitatio Anatomica de motu Cordis et sanguinis in animalbus* (Frankfurt, 1628), a poorly printed book of seventy pages (with two additional pages of errata), gave the first clear demonstration of the way to verification in the natural sciences, by careful observation and analysis of a phenomenon, the formulation of a tentative explanation for it, the devising of quantitative testing of the hypothesis and conclusions based on the results of the experiments.

In regard to drug use, Harvey indicated that drugs taken by mouth were absorbed into the blood stream from the gastro-enteric tract and distributed by the blood to various parts of the body on which they might act.

This idea was extended, after the gradual acceptance of Harvey's ideas, by Johann Sigmund Elscholtz (1623-1688), in the direct injection of drug solutions intravenously *(Clysmatica nova,* Berlin,

1665). He also undertook blood transfusion from dogs to dogs, and even from humans to humans. Blood transfusion from animal to animal was also accomplished by the keen Londoner, Richard Lower (1631-1691). Blood transfusions were tried clinically, but difficulties arose with unexplainable deaths. The procedure was banned legally in France and generally was abandoned. It was not revived until the twentieth century, after Karl Landsteiner (1868-1943) had described the iso-agglutinins which cause incompatibilities between the blood of differently grouped people *(Zbl Bact, 27:357-362, 1900)*.

A new feature of seventeenth century scientific effort was the establishment of scientific societies and systematic reporting of new scientific discoveries. The *Acadamia dei Lincei* flourished in Rome, and a group of young experimenters met in London and Oxford. This invisible college was chartered by Charles II in 1662 as the Royal Society of London for Promoting Natural Knowledge. The Academie des Sciences was founded in Paris by Louis XIV in 1666. The most influential was the Royal Society, thanks to the devoted enthusiasm, skill and persistence of its secretary, the Bremen linguistic theologian, Henry Oldenburg (1617-1677). He edited the first twelve volumes of its *Philosophical Transactions,* beginning in 1664, and obtained reports on all kinds of scientific activity from all over Europe.

It was here that Lower published his transfusion experiments *(Philos Trans, 3:226-232, 1666)*, and here his many friends reported on their studies. Among them were the great architect, Sir Christopher Wren (1632-1723) and the pioneer chemist, the Hon. Robert Boyle (1627-1691). Wren and Boyle collaborated on a study of the effects of the intravenous injections in dogs of solutions of opium and of crocus metallorum. The latter was prepared by igniting antimony metal with potassium nitrate to yield liver of antimony, which, when treated with water, gave crocus metallorum, a mixture of antimony oxides. Here was a beginning of direct pharmacological experimentation with new chemical substances.

Wren practically rebuilt London after the disastrous fire of 1665. His architectural genius is cherished in the parish churches of London and in St. Paul's cathedral. In 1696 he designed the simple main building of the College of William and Mary in Williamsburg, Virginia, where a fine full-length portrait of Boyle hangs. In 1661 London had a population of 460,000, as reported by John Grant (1620-1674), pioneer medical statistician.

Boyle's major claim to fame was his discovery of the inverse relation between the volume and pressure of gases, and his invention of suction pumps by which air could be withdrawn from a bell jar. With this instrument he showed that air is necessary both for life and for combustion, thus starting the successful search for what we call oxygen.

Boyle was an ingenious experimenter and cautious as well, as is clear in his *The Skeptical Chemist* (London, 1661), which was a sharp crack at the popular Paracelsians. In his *History of Human Blood* (London, 1683/4), he began an analysis of blood and of wine from the standpoint of their physicochemical properties, thus helping to begin physiological chemistry. He attempted a definition of chemical elements, and he first isolated acetone. In his *Specifick Medicines* (London, 1685), Boyle does not follow his scientific standard, but, writing from memory, refers chiefly to worn-out conventional formulations.

Another brilliant Fellow of the young Royal Society was John Mayo (1643-1679). He showed that dark venous blood becomes red by taking something from air, which is also a constituent of niter (KNO_3), and that this nitro-aer is supplied to foeti through maternal blood. Further, he localized the source of animal heat in muscles. His *Tractatus Quinque Medico-physici* (Oxford, 1747) is a rare medical classic.

Of greater interest to the history of pharmacology was Thomas Willis (1621-1675), a popular London practitioner who gave clear pioneering clinical descriptions of myasthenia gravis, of puerperal fever, and of diabetes mellitus. His *Pharmaceutica Rationalis* (London, 1647) aided in removing many complex and worn-out drug mixtures from the pharmacopeias. A great step in this direction was given by the critical London clinician, William Heberden (1710-1801), in his devastating attack on the almost superstitious use of two ancient mixtures in his *Essay on Mithradatium and Theriaka* (London, 1745).

By the eighteenth century, thanks in large part to the impact of Isaac Newton (1642-1727) and his *Principia* (London, 1687), the general idea of law and order in the universe was firmly established. This led inevitably to the successful classification of physical objects, including living things, but not to medical concepts. With no verifiable etiology for infectious or metabolic disorders, there could be no satisfactory nosology: symptoms of disease were nonspecific and variable.

The classification of living things, plants and animals, was brilliantly achieved by Carl Linné (1707-1778) in his *Systema Naturae* (Leyden, 1735). This went into many editions, of which the tenth in 1758 systematized the specific names for living things. The sources of drugs, plant, animal and mineral could now satisfactorily be identified, and their natural relations recognized. This was what made it possible for Charles Darwin (1809-1882) to carry through his remarkable study of natural selections with species evolution and adaptive survival.

Concern with the identification of plant remedies led many alert physicians in the seventeenth century to study botany. In 1670 a physic garden was established in Edinborough, and in 1679 a botanic garden was founded in Berlin. The famed Royal Botannic Gardens, at Kew in London, were not in use until 1730, but an herb garden was functioning in Madrid in 1718 and in St. Petersburg in 1713.

Fungus diseases of plants was first noted in 1677 by Robert Hooke (1635-1703), the skilled English microscopist who first defined cells in his *Micrographia* (J. Martyn, London, 1665). The most notorious of plant fungi is ergot, *Claviceps purpurea*, the cause of St. Anthony's Fire, the epidemic ergotism resulting from bread made from smutty grain.

In trying, in 1695, to analyze the health giving waters at Epsom Spa, Nehemia Grew (1641-1712), a keen physician botanist, isolated epsom salts (magnesium sulfate), a useful saline purge. Grew was the first to note pollen grains and the first to undertake a systematic anatomical analysis of plants. Friedrich Hoffman (1660-1742) introduced Seidlitz Powders, a mixture of magnesium and sodium sulfates, from a mineral spring in Seidlitz, Bohemia. Hoffman, in describing chlorosis, recommended a meat diet for its control. He also introduced an alcoholic opium preparation, Hoffman's Anodyne, for pain relief.

A number of pharmacological items of interest may be noted chronologically as they were noted in the first half of the eighteenth century. The Apothecaries Company of London was founded in 1721, and immediately set about to establish appropriate guidelines for the collection, preservation, preparation and dispensing of the many crude drugs available. In 1732, Thomas Dover (1660-1742), the buccaneering physician who rescued Alexander Selkirk (Robinson Crusoe) from the island of Juan Fernandes, introduced his diaphoretic powder of opium and ipecac in his formulary entitled *An Ancient Physician's Legacy to His Country*. Dover's Powder has been used into our own time for the purpose of aborting a cold.

In 1733, the Rev. Stephen Hales (1677-1761), who first directly measured blood pressure in an obliging old mare, produced dropsy in her by injecting water intravenously. In 1736, the great Swiss physiologist, Albrecht von Haller (1708-1777) showed that bile is necessary for the digestion of fat. His theory of irritability and his direct demonstration overthrew the Galenical-scholastic idea that nerves carry a fluid, thus opening a path to neurophysiology and neuropharmacology. In 1739 Percival Pott (1714-1788), who described chimney-sweep's cancer of the scrotum, first recommended bismuth ointments for skin lesions. Mention should also be made of the great Swedish chemist, Carl Wilhelm Scheele (1742-1786), a pharmacist who described calcium phosphate in bone, discovered hydrogen sulfide, oxygen, chlorine, and tartaric, gallic, oxalic, citric, lactic and malic acids. He recognized the toxic properties of some of these compounds. As an amusing sidelight, it should be noted that in 1747, the Massachusetts Colony passed an act designed to stop pollution of Boston Harbor.

Pharmacopeias were far more important in the eighteenth century than now. Both physicians and apothecaries relied on pharmacopeias as a major source of information on drugs, especially the newly introduced ones. Prescriptions were carefully devised and prepared in accordance with the judgment of the physician and the skill of the pharmacist for each individual patient. The first London Pharmacopeia of 1618 contained many traditional mixtures

Drugs in the Seventeenth and Eighteenth Centuries

and much actual filth. The fourth edition of 1721, compiled by Hans Sloane (1660-1753), whose library became the nucleus of the British Museum, introduced stramonium, ipecac, tartar emetic, iron sulfate and lime water, but still retained much trash. The fifth London Pharmacopeia of 1746 dropped unicorn horn, spider webs and virgin's milk, but mithridate, theriac, and bezoars were retained, while Glauber's salts and sweet spirits of nitre were added. Heberden's expose of mithridate and theriac led to their omission from the sixth edition in 1788. Added at this time were castor oil, quassia, zinc oxide, compound tincture of benzoin, and tincture opii camphorata or paregoric. This edition of the London Pharmacopeia, and the one of 1809 which included digitalis, set the example for the first U.S. Pharmacopeia of 1820.

One of the unpleasant aspects of the long sea voyages undertaken during the Renaissance and with increasing frequency in the seventeenth and eighteenth centuries was scurvy. This was a serious disease afflicting the sailors and often resulting in incapacity or death. It was slowly recognized that scurvy was due to the restricted diet common on long voyages. Although seemingly recognized from antiquity, it wasn't until the sixteenth century that effective means were found to treat or prevent the scorbutus.

The first to report a successful remedy was Jacques Cartier (1491-1557), the French explorer of the St. Lawrence Valley in Canada. In the winter of 1535, his men and the neighboring natives suffered severely, with many deaths from pestilence which must have been scurvy. A native told how a decoction of bark and leaves from a certain tree had cured him. The story is well told by B. Holmsted and G. Liljestrand *(Readings in Pharmacology,* Oxford, 1963). According to them, the tree was indentified as arbor vitae, *Thuja occidentalis,* an evergreen tree indigenous to northeast North America. The leaves and bark contain thuja ($C_{20}H_{22}O_{12}$), a glucoside which resembles quercetrin and which has antiscorbutic properties.

The use of oranges and lemons to cure scurvy was first described by Baldiunus Ronsaeus (1525-1597) in his tract on scorbuto (Antwerp, 1564), and John Woodall (1556-1643), surgeon to St. Bartholomew's Hospital, London, recommended their use for seamen in *The Surgeons Mate* (London, 1617). The leaves and barks of many North American trees continued in popular use as antiscorbutics for many decades. In my seventeenth century family recipe book is a formula for "A best drink for the scurvy" which includes two ounces each of sassafras, sarsaparilla and hartshorn leaves to six gallons of yeast brew. This seems to have been prepared for use on sea voyages. Sassafras contains a tannin derivative, with a volatile oil made up largely of safrol, the methylene ether of allyl pyrocatechol. This is a toxic hypotensive agent. Sassafras oil also contains pinene, a skin irritating terpene. Pine oils were recommended to Cook as antiscorbutics by Linne. Sarsaparilla contains glucosides, such as sarsasaponin ($C_{22}H_{36}O_{10}$). The use of decoctions of sarsaparilla was probably a folklore hangover of its presumed power as a blood-purifier.

It was in the seventeenth and eighteenth centuries, however, that antiscorbutics became more widely known. In his *Rarioum plantarum historia* (Amsterdam, 1601), Carl Chisius (1524-1609), the Leyden botanist, describes the excellent antiscorbutic properties of cloud berries *(Rubus chamaemous)*, related to blackberries and raspberries. The fruit was made into jellies by the Scandinavians and used successfully in treating scurvy. Ascorbic acid has been found in such fruits.

The eventual eradication of scurvy from seamen was due to the persistent efforts of James Lind (1716-1794), founder of naval hygiene, to get the British Navy to provide lime, lemon or orange juices regularly to sailors at sea. James Cook (1728-1779), the great Pacific explorer, demonstrated the success of Lind's recommendations, and in spite of occasional jibes, British sailors were glad to be called "limeys."

Characteristic of seventeenth and eighteenth century science was the slow and blundering attempts to develop quantitative methodology. This probably stemmed from the successful physical measurements introduced by Galileo Galilei (1564-1642), son of a physician, and professor in the Medical Faculty at Padua. Harvey probably studied under him and derived quantitative ideas in experimentation from him. One of his colleagues was Santonio Santorio (1561-1636) who first measured water metabolism in experiments on himself suspended in a steelyard balance. Probably also under the dawning influence of quantitation was Regner de Graaf (1641-1673) who measured the rate of secretion from the pancreatic gland in dogs after devising a successful pancreatic fistula. He also measured salivary secretion, as well as biliary secretion.

Systematic experimentation with drugs developed slowly. In 1676, Johannes Wepfer (1620-1695) demonstrated nux vomica tetanus *(Strychnos nux vomica)* in dogs, and showed toxic effects of tobacco *(Nicotiana tobacum)* and of water hemlock *(Conium verpa)*. From these crude preparations were later to be isolated the active principles, the alkaloids called respectively strychnine, nicotine and coniine. These early experiments helped in characterizing the biological activities of the crude preparations for recognition of their toxic properties. Crude dosage quantitation, even of unstandardized preparations, could give some indication of what to expect from varying dosage.

Similar experiments were made by Anton Storck (1731-1803) on hemlock (conium), stramonium (jimson weed from Virginia; *Datura stramonium*), aconite (monkshood, wolfsbane; *Aconitum napellus*), and hyoscyamus (henbane: *Hyoscyamus niger*), These experiments cleared the way for later attempts to isolate the respective active principles, free from the tannins, gums and other extraneous material,—the alkaloids: coniine, atropine, aconitine, and hyoscyamine with hyoscine or scopolamine.

Felice Fontana (1730-1805) extended his careful and detailed pioneering studies on effects of snake venoms in various animals and birds including plant drugs. He concluded from a vast number of experiments that the general symptoms of drug action are due to particular effects on specific organs. Fontana's wide-ranging studies, which kept him in contact with the best biomedical scholars of his time, are being explored for definitive analysis by my long-time colleague, Peter K. Knoefel, of Firenze.

The quantitative experimental approach was especially successful in developing modern chemistry, and thus in making a firm foundation for pharmacological study of pure chemical substances. This chemical effort followed Boyle's technical success in handling gases. It is interesting that Boyle should have been a leader in developing a corpuscular theory of matter in opposition to the Paracelsians who held to a vague essence permeating matter. The word gas, which Boyle made scientifically respectable, had been invented by Jean Baptiste van Helmont (1577-1644), a leading Paracelsian, to designate the spiritous essence coming forth from fermentation or putrefaction.

Thanks to the technical advances made by Boyle, study on gases proceeded vigorously in the latter part of the eighteenth century. The first truly modern chemist was the shrewd Scot, Joseph Black (1728-1799), who overthrew the phlogiston theory of the Bavarian, George Ernest Stahl (1660-1734). Stahl considered heat or phlogiston to be a substance. Thus a typical example used for teaching was that when lime-stone or powdered lime was heated, it gained phlogiston, and that when quick lime was slaked with water, it lost phlogiston. Black showed that heated lime loses "fixed air," as he called it, carbon dioxide as we say, according to our notation: $CaCO_3 = CaO + CO_2$. On the other hand, Black showed that quicklime, when slaked, gains something: $CaO + H_2O = Ca(OH)_2$. This fixed air, coming from heated limestone, Black also found in expired air of mammals. He noted that it does not support respiration, but is not actually toxic *(Dissertatio medical inauguralis de mumore acidis a cibo orto,* Edinburgh, 1854). As Garrison says, "Thus Black had again isolated the carbonic acid gas which van Helmont had, over a hundred years before, noted in fermentation as *gas sylvestre."* Black also described nitrogen, which he called azote.

Then came that Birmingham clergyman, Joseph Priestley (1733-1804) to mess matters up again. Priestley isolated what we called oxygen, but which he thought of as dephlogisticated air, for he was caught in the trap of Stahl's phlogiston. Although he noted that plants restore viated air, he thought that respiration involved the phlogistication of dephlogisticated air. How foolish this now seems to be! Priestly also made nitrous oxide (Observations on Different Kinds of Air, *Phil Trans Lond, 62*:147-264, 1772), but did not experiment with it. Suspected later of sympathizing with the French revolutionaries, a mob burned his home and he fled to Pennsylvania. He settled on the Susquehanna River and resumed his chemical studies. The American Chemical Society maintains his home as a museum, thanks to the prodding of Edgar Fahs Smith (1856-1928), the great chemist of the University of Pennsylvania.

The facts about respiratory gaseous exchange were revealed by the quantitative chemical methods introduced by Antoine-Laurent Lavoisier (1743-1794). He also discovered oxygen and named it *(Hist Acad R Sci,* Paris, 1778). He demonstrated that oxygen is removed from air during respiration and that carbon dioxide is added in proportion to the oxygen used. Meanwhile, iron had been shown to be present in blood, but its relation to oxygen transport was not revealed until hemoglobin was discovered and analyzed at a later time.

These metabolic experiments were carefully conducted with quantitative estimates of the gases used or evolved. Lavoisier's wife kept the records as contemporary sketch records. Lavoisier was guillotined because, being Director of the Mint, he was suspected of coin-clipping. His widow married the U.S.A. Tory, Benjamin Thompson, Count Rumford (1753-1814), who explored the mechanical equivalent of heat. The steam engine had long before been invented by Thomas Newcomen (1603-1729) with reciprocating governing control added in 1765 by James Watt (1736-1819).

While Lavoisier had thought that the oxidation of carbon occurs in the lungs, the great physicist Joseph Louis Lagrange (1736-1813), who worked with Lavoisier, corrected this error. His pupil, Jean Henri Hassenfratz (1775-1827) indicated that the oxygen in the blood from inspired air slowly takes up carbon and hydrogen from organic compounds in tissues as blood moves through them. Henry Cavendish (1731-1810) had already isolated hydrogen and showed the composition of air. The facts were finally demonstrated when Henrick Gustav Magnus (1802-1870) quantitatively analyzed blood gases, showing that arterial blood gives up oxygen to tissues, whereupon venous blood takes up carbon dioxide from tissues. Thus, finally the "fuliginous vapors" of Galenical tradition which had puzzled Harvey were explained.

This extensive study of respiratory gases greatly stimulated medical interest. Thomas Beddoes (1760-1808) of Shropshire founded the Pneumatic Institute in Clifton in 1798 for treatment of disease by inhalation of gases. His apparatus was made by James

Watt who invented a gasometer. His Director of Research was the brilliant Humphrey Davy (1778-1829) who described the anesthetic action of nitrous oxide in experiment on himself.

Davy recommended its use to relieve pain in surgery but there were no takers *(Researches, chemical and philosophical, chiefly concerning nitrous oxide,* London, 1800). He postulated that heat is a form of motion, and went on to study the effects of electric currents on solutions of salts, and isolated sodium, potassium, boron, calcium, magnesium, strontium, barium, and chlorine. Suggesting that hydrogen is responsible for acidity, he showed the electronegative character of iodine and chlorine, and invented the Davy safety lamps for miners which are still used.

It was thus, with sparkling chemical achievement, that the path was opened for the full theoretical and practical development of pharmacology in the nineteenth century. Now with precise analytical methods in chemistry, the composition of crude drug preparations, many used from antiquity, could be investigated. Now quantitative methods were becoming available for the measurement of functional activity, including drug effects. Soon would come methods of synthesis for new drugs, hopefully safer and more specifically effective in disease than those found in nature. Protopharmacology led into real pharmacology at the close of the eighteenth century.

CHAPTER 9

THE FIRST PART OF THE NINETEENTH CENTURY

A desire to take medicine is, perhaps, the great feature which distinguishes people from other animals.

WILLIAM OSLER (1849-1919)
Science, 17:170, 1891

THE BASIC TECHNIQUES OF chemical analysis which had been introduced toward the end of the eighteenth century were first successfully applied to pharmacology by Friedrich Wilhelm Adam Sertürner (1783-1841), a pharmacist from Paderborn in Westphalia. As a young man he was interested in opium, and in 1805 he described the isolation of meconic acid from the crude extract of opium. In 1806, he extracted opium with acid, obtaining a water soluble substance precipitated as white crystals by ammonia. This showed it to be a weak base. Experimenting with it on dogs, Sertürner found it causes sleep and indifference to pain, so he recognized it as the "specific narcotic substance" of opium. Going on with his studies, Sertürner called this new substance morphine in honor of the Graeco-Roman god of sleep, Morpheus. His studies included experiments on himself and three of his friends. They ingested about ten times the now recommended dosage of morphine; it had a profound depressant reaction from which they recovered in a few days. Sertürner's report (*Ann Physik,* 25:56-89, 1817) attracted wide attention, and his chemical technique was promptly applied to many other well-known crude drugs.

There was some controversy about the isolation of morphine.

Louis Charles Derosné (1780-1846) isolated crystals from opium in 1804, but failed to characterize them and did not realize that they may have been the chief biologically active agent in opium. The same comment applies to the work of Armand Seguin (1767-1835), published in 1814. Derosné was responsible for developing beet sugar. Seguin was a pupil of Lavoisier and studied the precipitation of what we call protein in the tanning process, either with tannin or metallic salts.

K. F. W. Meissner (1792-1853) of Halle gave the name alkaloid (alkali-like) to those weak bases obtained from crude drug sources by Sertürner's method. With Joseph Bienaimé Caventou (1795-1877), he isolated veratrine in 1818 from seeds of hellebore *(Schoen ocaulon officinali* or the American Veratrium Viride). Hellebore was known from antiquity as an irritating poison. Veratrine is now known to be a mixture of several related alkaloids, the chief one being veratradine. The tincture of Veratrum was long used as a local irritant and as a hypotensive agent. In 1819, Meissner and Caventou isolated colchicine ($C_{22}H_{25}NO_6$) from the corm of *Colchicum autummale,* the autumn crocus, used from Roman times in treating gout. For this it remains helpful. It also causes doubling of chromosomes and is used in genetic research.

Caventou was professor of toxicology in the Pharmacy School of Paris. Here he joined Pierre Joseph Pelletier (1788-1842) in a series of brilliant alkaloidal discoveries. Both were greatly influenced by the chemical techniques expounded by Claude Louis Berthollet (1748-1822) and Joseph Gay-Lussac (1778-1850). Berthollet worked with Lavoisier in devising a workable chemical nomenclature, discovered chlorine bleach, and developed the principle of mass action. The happy traveler, Gay-Lussac, outlined the principles of chemical combination of elements.

In quick order, Caventou and Pelletier isolated strychnine from *nux vomica* in 1818; the very poisonous brucine in 1819, and also from seeds of *Strychnos nux vomica,* and caffeine from coffee beans in 1821. Their great achievement, however, was to isolate quinine from cinchona bark in 1820. This quickly became the favored remedy for all fevers, and, with increasing shortage of natural supplies, led to amazingly successful attempts to find synthetic substitutes. Caventou and Pelletier were devoted scientific friends. A bronze statue in their honor, standing together, was erected in front of the Ecole de Pharmacie. It was destroyed by the Nazis.

Pelletier isolated narceine and thebaine from opium in 1832 and 1833 respectively, with Jean Baptiste André Dumas (1800-1884). Dumas was a keen young chemist who studied iodine compounds for treatment of goiter, who found anthracene, and made methyl alcohol in 1834. Friedlieb Ferdinand Runge (1795-1867) of Breslau isolated caffeine from coffee also in 1821. He went on to prepare phenol, and found pyrrole and aniline in coal tar in 1834. He also pioneered in the now popular paper chromatography. Pierre Jean Robiquet (1780-1840) isolated narcotine from opium in 1817, and codeine in 1833.

Philipp Lounz Geiger (1785-1836) of Heidelberg, with his pupil, Germain Henri Hess (1802-1850), later in St. Petersburg, isolated atropine from belladonna leaves *(Atropa belladonna)* known from antiquity for dilating the pupil and relieving asthma; aconitine from *Aconitum napellus* and other poisonous Ranunculaceac known from antiquity; colchicine from autumn crocus; coniine, or propylpiperidine from *Conium maculata,* which Socrates drank in his civilized self-execution at the will of the Athenians, and hyoscyamine from henbane *(Hyoscyamus niger,* and also from *Atropa belladonna* and *Datura stramonium* or Jamestown, Jimson weed). The brilliant work of Geiger and Hess was reported in 1833.

To indicate the discovery of other important alkaloids, it may be noted that Georg Franz Merck (1825-1873) described papaverine from opium *(Liebig's Ann, 73:*50-55, 1950). This led him to develop his family's seventeenth century Angel Apothecary in Darmstadt into a major alkaloid supply concern. Later this led to the brilliant expansion of Merck and Company in Rahway, New Jersey, an outstanding industrial drug producer, especially of vitamins, antibiotics, and many synthetics tailored to specification.

Albert Niemann (1840-1921) isolated cocaine from coca leaves in 1860 as a young student of Friedrich Wöhler (1800-1882). It was Wöhler who had isolated the elements aluminum and beryllium in 1827 and 1828, and who had demolished the distinction between inorganic and organic (or vital, living) chemistry by synthesizing urea, a typical animal product of presumed little biological activity, from ammonium cyanate, a typical inorganic compound, (*Ann Phys Chem, 12*:253-256, 1828). With Justus von Liebig (1803-1873) of Darmstadt, Wöhler in 1837 had isolated amygdalin (mandelo-nitryl glucoside, from seeds of *Rosaceae*, especially almonds), and had prepared hydroquinone in 1848. Liebig, who had a pioneer student chemical laboratory, synthesized chloroform and chloral hydrate in 1831, studied uric acid and hippuric acid formation in the body, classified foods as fats, carbohydrates and proteins, and demonstrated the carbon and nitrogen cycles between plants and animals.

Most fruitful for pharmacology was Pelletier's association with the handsome, brilliant and independent François Magendie (1783-1855). They isolated emetine in 1822 from ipecac *(Uragoga ipecacuanha)* and named it in relation to its marked emetic activity. This led Magendie to a critical and classic study of the physiology of swallowing and vomiting. He normally found sugar in mammalian blood, and demonstrated that ventral spinal nerves have a motor action while the dorsal spinal nerves carry peripheral sensory stimuli into the central nervous system. This was clearly demonstrated by Magendie by 1822, although the artistic anatomist Charles Bell (1774-1842) of Edinburgh had made the same observation about a year previously. Professor J. M. D. Olmsted thought that Magendie deserves the credit *(François Magendie,* New York 1944).

As early as 1809, Magendie was studying the Borneo arrow poison, *Upas tiente,* a member of the *Strychnos* genus related to *Apocinae*. It is a powerful convulsant. Using dogs and even horses, he tried to localize the pathways of absorption and distribution, as well as the place of action. Water or alcoholic preparations of nux vomica and St. Ignatius bean were found to have the same effects as *upas*.

By 1821, Magendie was sufficiently impressed by the importance of the newly discovered alkaloids to issue his famed *Formu-*

laire pour la préparation at l'emploi de plusiers nouveaux medicaments (Paris, 1821), in which he described the actions and indicated chemical uses for morphine, prussic acid, strychnine, quinine, emetine, iodine, and other chemical compounds, organic and inorganic. This classic formulary went into nine editions, with many translations, and established pharmacology as the basis for a rational drug therapy derived from direct observation and experimentation rather than from theory.

Actually Magendie and his pupils at the College de France did lay the foundations for the modern science of pharmacology by clearly outlining the fundamental scientific problems with which pharmacology is concerned, and which are not within the scope of any other scientific discipline. These are: 1) the dose-effect relationships, qualitatively explored from antiquity, but not quantitated satisfactorily until 1927, when the London mathematician, J. W. Trevan (1887-1955) showed the Gaussian distribution of variation in the graded response of living material to the same dose of a drug; 2) factors, both time and chemical, involved in the absorption, distribution, chemical transformation, and removal of drugs into and out of living material, a study formalized and extended by Oswald Schmiedeberg (1838-1921), J. Von Mering (1849-1908), and Marcel Von Nencki (1847-1901); 3) the localization of the site of action of a drug, first explored by Claude Bernard (1813-1878), Magendie's pupil, in demonstrating that the muscular paralyzing effect of curare is due to its block of nerve impulse transmission at the neuromuscular junction; 4) the specific mechanism of the action of a drug, again first demonstrated by Claude Bernard in showing that the effects of carbon monoxide are due to its irreversible combination with hemoglobin so that oxygen cannot be carried to tissues, so that tissue asphyxiation occurs, and 5) the relation between the chemical constitution of a drug and its biological activity (biochemorphology or structure-action relation), first and brilliantly explored by another pupil of Magendie's, James Blake (1814-1893), for inorganic salts, and later by A. C. Brown (1839-1923) and T. R. Fraser (1841-1920) of Edinburgh for nitrogen containing organic compounds.

Here is the clear beginning of modern pharmacology. Under Magendie's guidance Bernard, Blake, and Magendie himself laid the broad foundations for all the complex scientific studies of drug development and action and the application of this knowledge to a wide variety of professional and social problems.

A frustrated tragic dramatist, Claude Bernard was inspired by Magendie and extended the experimental method to encompass physiology and medicine as well as pharmacology. He followed Magendie at the College de France. He investigated fat and carbohydrate digestion, discovered the glycogenic function of the liver, and demonstrated nervous control of local blood supply. His most important contribution was his idea of a *milieu interieur,* an internal steady state whereby various functional buffers adjust to various stresses in order to preserve physiological constancy. This was later expanded by Walter B. Cannon (1871-1945) to the concept of homeostasis. Under the mathematical guidance of Norbert Wiener (1894-1964) and the idea of feedback control, it became part of computer technology, thanks to John von Neumann (1903-1957). A handsome heroic bronze statue of Claude Bernard was erected in front of the College de France. This was destroyed by the Nazis.

In addition to his classic pharmacological studies on the mechanism of action of carbon monoxide and on the site of action of curare, Bernard made many careful studies on the action of anesthetic agents. He well distinguished between asphyxia or anoxia and anesthesia. His was the first experimental theory of the mechanism of anesthesia: reversible coagulation of proteins in nerves and muscles. Bernard, although publishing reports on his searches and researches as he went along, admirably summarized them in a famed series of lectures. As his biographer, James M. D. Olmsted says. (*Claude Bernard, Physiologist,* New York, 1938) he fashioned his careful lectures on those of Magendie, and in spite of his dramatic flair, he was easily distracted by feminine listeners.

Of chief interest to pharmacologists are Bernard's *Leçons sur les effets des substances toxiques et medicamentouses* (Paris, 1857), and his *Leçons sur les anesthesiques et sur l'asphyxie* (Paris, 1875). As early as 1855 Bernard was experimenting with chloroform and curare. His scientific findings appeared in the current scientific journals after presentation at a meeting, quite as we do today.

In the 1858 lectures on toxic substances, Bernard offered a fine eulogy to Magendie, with a bibliography. These lectures contained descriptions of the analyzed gaseous content of blood and a full account of the mechanism of toxicity of carbon monoxide. He demonstrated that the lethal effects of carbon monoxide are due to an irreversible combination with hemoglobin, thus preventing adequate transport of oxygen to tissues. There are discussions on asphyxiation and artificial respiration. In a clear account of curare, after an historical introduction, there is the demonstration that the drug causes muscular paralysis by blocking the transmission of nerve impulses to muscles. After consideration of the poisonous actions of strychnine, venoms, and nicotine, Bernard discussed the toxicity of alcohol, ether, and chloroform. He noted their interference with pancreatic and intestinal secretions and with liver function. Ether, he suggested, renders an animal diabetic, probably by disturbing the glycogenic function of the liver. This was one of his great discoveries.

In his lectures on anesthetic agents, Bernard returned to his early studies on chloroform, in which he had suggested a theory for general anesthesia. He did not believe that asphyxia plays much of a part in actual anesthesia, although he fully recognized its dangers during anesthesia. By 1870, however, asphyxia was usually thought to be the chief causal factor of anesthesia. It may have been this which persuaded Bernard to offer a series of lectures on anesthesia where he reviewed his experiments of a couple decades earlier. Bernard sharply criticized the asphyxia theory of anesthesia, and proposed one based on his studies with chloroform.

Bernard was a skilled experimenter, and was accustomed to working on isolated neuromuscle preparations, as in his studies with curare. When he applied chloroform to muscle, he found that it lost excitability and gradually became rigid and opaque. If the concentration of chloroform wasn't too great, Bernard found that washing the chloroform away with physiological salt solution would restore the nerves and muscles to their usual condition so that they would again conduct impulses and contract. He seems to have noted similar results with ether and alcohol. He proposed that anesthesia was due to a reversible coagulation of the chemical constituents of nerves and muscles, chiefly proteins.

Bernard's theory of anesthesia was promptly criticized on the grounds that a higher concentration of an anesthetic agent was necessary to cause coagulation than that which would cause anesthesia. However, years later an effort was made to revive Bernard's reversible protein coagulation theory of anesthesia. W. D. Bancroft (1867-1953) and G. H. Richter of Cornell showed that low concentrations of volatile anesthetics produce reversible coagulation in various colloidal systems, even in yeast cells (*Proc Natl Acad Sci, 16*:573-577, 1930). However, Bancroft's experimental evidence was weak and he was generally suspected of wishful thinking. This was quite the antithesis of Claude Bernard's rigorous self-criticism. Yet, Bernard's theory of anesthesia was conclusively shown to be untenable in a careful study by V. E. Henderson (1877-1945) and G. H. W. Lucas of Toronto, who were well respected for their scientific work on anesthesia which resulted in the development of cyclopropane.

Actually, Claude Bernard's theory was generalized for narcosis. He realized that there are progressive stages in central nervous system depression from analgesia through anesthesia to coma. It was in connection with his broad concept of narcosis that Bernard suggested premedication with morphine before anesthetization, in order to reduce the amount of inhalation anesthetic agent required for satisfactory anesthesia. This was specifically spelled out by L. Labbé (1832-1916) for surgical use (*Compt Rend Acad Sci, 74*:627-29, 1872). Bernard had noted in 1864 that morphine potentiates chloroform activity. This led him to suggest premedication with morphine before inducing anesthesia. French surgeons generally adopted this procedure. This led to the use of atropine to counteract morphine depression and then to give atropine to prevent the vagal effects of chloroform on the heart. As Henderson later showed (*Physiol Rev, 10*:171-220, 1930), no satisfactory general theory for anesthesia has yet been proposed.

As Bernard suspected, it may be a phenomenon in which many factors are operative, and thus toward which many causes may contribute.

Magendie's other great but unrecognized pupil was James Blake, son of a dissenting brewing family in Gosport, England. Studying at University College, London, under such geniuses as the pioneer histologist, William Sharpey (1802-1880), and Thomas Graham (1805-1869), the founder of colloid chemistry, Blake was also greatly influenced by the chemical ideas of Humphrey Davy, John Dalton (1766-1844), who developed the atomic theory of the elements, and Michael Faraday (1791-1867), who founded electrochemistry. In the summers of 1838 and 1839, while a medical student at University College, Blake went to Paris and seems to have studied with Magendie. Bernard was a student there also. Blake must have been an acute observer. He was impressed by new technical procedures for the quantitative estimation of functional activity, such as blood pressure. In particular, he saw the advantages of measuring blood pressure by the ingenious mercury hemodynamometer invented by Jean Leonard Marie Poiseuille (1799-1869). Blake was the first to use this instrument in England. Actually, blood pressure, in a gentle mare, had first been measured by the Rev. Stephen Hales (1677-1761), curate of Teddington, but nothing had resulted from his *Statical Essays, Containing Haemostaticks* (London, 1733). Blake used the hemodynamometer well.

In 1839, while still a medical student, Blake reported on studies of the effects of various solutions injected directly into the blood stream of dogs. He describes the gross action of water on blood infusion, the blood pressure response to respiratory variations (noted by Hales), and the effects of the intravenous or intra-arterial injections of various sodium and potassium salts, then of such recently isolated alkaloids as strychnine, coniine, and morphine, and of such crude drug infusions as tobacco and digitalis. Noting the time interval between injection and the appearance of any functional change, such as respiratory or cardiac rate or amplitude, blood pressure, gastro-enteric activity, or neuromuscular effect, Blake was the first to measure circulation time and to grasp the concept of target organs for drug action (*Edin Med Surg J, 51*:33-49, 1839).

Blake reported further experiments with various inorganic salts (*Arch Gen Med, 6*:289-300, Nov., 1839). Writing in French, he proposed that there must be a relation between the chemical composition of a drug, and its biological activity. He implied that this problem could better be studied by the use of chemicals, such as inorganic salts whose constitution was relatively better known than by using drugs and such as the newly found alkaloids whose chemical makeup was unknown. Soon Blake was a qualified surgeon and had a Pall Mall practice. He was a founder of the Chemical Society. His pharmacological studies were supported by a grant of sixty pounds a year from the British Association for the Advancement of Science. I think this was the first grant-in aid of scientific research.

By 1846 Blake's effort, reported to the British Association, had resulted in several remarkable conclusions: 1) the characteristic action of an inorganic compound is due more to the electropositive element therein than to the electronegative one; 2) if one arranges the elements by increasing order of atomic weight, using the same corresponding salt throughout, one finds that the intensity of biological activity increases with atomic weight, and 3) if one arranges the elements in order of increasing atomic weight, using the same corresponding salt throughout, one finds that similar biological responses reappear, so that the elements may be grouped into families on the basis of their biological actions. This grouping is a skeleton of the Periodic Table of the elements. Nothing, it would seem, could better justify Blake's faith that a relation between the chemical constitution of a compound and its biological activity exists than to find the beginning of the Periodic Table of the chemical elements in the results of the experiments he reported.

Later Blake modestly declined any anticipation of the demonstration of periodicity among the chemical elements, as made on strict physicochemical data by Dimitri Mendeleyev (1834-1907) of St. Petersburg in 1869. Actually Blake went on to claim from the results of his studies that the determining factor in the periodicity of biological action of inorganic salts is isomorphism or crystallizable configuration.

Blake's clinical skill was apparent from a note (*Lancet, 1:* 873-874, March 9, 1839) in which he suggested that mere scratching of the intima of a varicose vein by a needle would produce enough inflammation to close it as well as any sclerosing chemical. Clearly he was destined for a brilliant career in London. In 1847 he suddenly appeared in St. Louis as Professor of Anatomy and Surgery at the pioneering University of St. Louis. From here he published a summary of his experiments on the biological activity of inorganic salts (*Am J Med Sci, 15,* n.s. 63-76, Jan. 1848). Within three years Blake was going overland in the Gold Rush to California.

In Sacramento, Blake was a busy general practitioner and chemical assayer. When the *California Medical Journal* appeared in 1856, he contributed clinical essays and a remarkable discussion of the theory of probability. After the 1862 flood, Blake came to San Francisco as editor of the *Pacific Medical and Surgical Journal.* He quit this in disgust at the poor quality of contributions. Meanwhile he made a pioneering contribution to the open-air rest treatment for tuberculosis, asserting that this was vastly superior to any drug or other therapy (*Am J Med Sci, 46:* 323-330, 1863).

In San Francisco, Blake became Professor of Midwifery and Diseases of Women and Children at the University of California Medical School and acquired the reputation of being a practical clinician with no fancy scientific theorizing. As President of the newly formed California Academy of Science, Blake reported on his extensive studies in meterology (with prescience of the polar-front idea), in geology (with pioneer mapping of the Nevada Great Basin), in biochemistry (with cholesterol analyses of yolk sacs of ambiticoid fishes), and in many other scientific fields from archeology to zoology. He studied the composition of mineral waters and investigated the chemical composition both of soils and of grapes with regard to their fitness for making wine. As an example of applied agricultural pharmacology, he introduced the use of carbon bisulfide for killing the roundworms *(Phylloxera)* in the soil which did such damage to French vineyards. This was a pioneering development of an effective pest control.

In 1876 Blake suddenly left San Francisco to open a tuberculosis sanitarium east of Mount St. Helena. He ran this with a Mrs. Emaline Woods, a frontier character who wore pants, smoked a pipe, and "swore like a trooper."

In 1880 they moved to Middletown, a small place nearby. There Blake resumed his early studies on the biological action of inorganic salts. He now received samples of salts of rare earth from Sir William Crookes (1832-1919) who had discovered thallium in 1861. Blake's report was the first on the toxicity of its salts. Blake used a spectroscope to follow the rate of its urinary secretion. He noted increase in complexity of biological activity with increase in valence of metallic salts and reported his findings in German and French scientific journals as well as those in English. He took the long journey from California to Europe at least thrice in order to report on the results of his studies. On one meeting in the rooms of the Royal Society in Burlington House, London, he complained of finding it odd that a young man should report, as a new finding, the arteriolar constriction following digitalis, when he, Blake, had reported the same finding in that very room fifty years earlier.

Magendie and his pupils, Bernard and Blake, clearly established modern pharmacology. They outlined its characteristic scientific problems and they made remarkable contributions toward their tentative solution. Blake had no pupils. One of Bernard's greatest was Paul Bert (1833-1886), who discovered caisson disease, "the bends," caused by liberation of nitrogen bubbles in blood on release from pressure. Bert's studies on gaseous tensions in relation to respiration are basic for aviation or space physiology. He noted oxygen toxicity at high pressure and showed high altitude is due to anoxemia.

Magendie and his pupils were part of the brilliant Parisian medical group, which included François Joseph Victor Broussais (1772-1838); Pierre Alexander Louis (1787-1872); Rene-Théophile Hyacinthe Laennec (1781-1826), who invented stethescopes and rationalized diagnosis; Pierre Bretonneau (1771-1862), who outlined the germ theory of infectious disease; Phillippe Pinel (1745-1826), who started modern and humane psychiatry, and Philippe Ricord (1799-1889) who finally differentiated and clearly characterized the venereal diseases. This keen group attracted the best of the young physicians from the United States, including Oliver Wendell Holmes (1809-1894), long Professor of Anatomy at Harvard, and renowned for his wit, some of it against drug excesses; William Wood Gerhard (1809-1872), who differentiated typhus and typhoid fevers, and Ashbel Smith (1805-1886) who founded the University of Texas.

Broussais and Louis are especially interesting for a history of applied pharmacology. Broussais was the last of the Galenical humoralists. Believing in heroic efforts to abort disease, he used large doses of purgatives and emetics, and copious bleeding. He used leeches for bleeding, sometimes applying a dozen or more. This sort of violent therapy had caused ridicule in England. One of its chief proponents had been John Lettsom (1744-1815). He was satirized in the doggerel:

> When my patients come to me,
> I physicks, bleeds and sweats 'em"
> And if then, they go and die,
> What's that to me: I Lettsom.

Yet, he had given in his account of chronic alcoholism a pioneering description of drug addiction *(Mem Med Soc Lond, 1:*128-165, 1779-87).

Broussais' violent therapy was demolished by the statistical evidence of Louis. He showed by rigid control studies of the untreated in comparison with patients who were bled by Broussais' method, that in pneumonia the untreated patients had less distress or mortality than those who had been treated. Similarly he disproved the use of the inhalation of chlorine gas in treating respiratory disease.

Somewhat the same statistical technique resulted in the conquest of puerperal fever, the dread disease which made childbirth a horror in the first half of the nineteenth century. Oliver Wendell Holmes in 1843 had reported on the contagiousness of puerperal fever but was jeered for his effort and did nothing further. However, Ignaz Philipp Semmelweis (1818-1865) did. Semmelweis noticed a difference in the mortality rates of lying-in women in two different wards of the Allgemeines Krankenhaus in Vienna: In a teaching ward, where an effort was made at cleanliness, deaths were fewer than in the other where students came from the dissecting room and without washing their hands, undertook vaginal examination before delivery. Semmelweis noted that the symptoms and pathological lesions in puerperal fevers were the same as those displayed by a colleague who died of a dissection wound. Semmelweis required all who attended the lying-in women to wash their hands in a solution of calcium chloride before entering the wards. Promptly, within a year, the mortality fell from 9.9 percent to 1.2 percent. Semmelweis was jeered and retired to teach in Budapest. He was the pioneer in the use of antiseptics in surgery and obstetrics (*Die Aetiologie, der Bergriff, und die Prophylaxis des Kindbettfiebers,* Budapest, 1861).

Another great advance in making modern surgery and obstetrics possible was anesthesia, a practical contribution developed by practical means in the vigorously practical United States. This story begins with the Philadelphia reaction to Humphrey Davy's 1800 account of nitrous oxide and its biological effects. In 1808, William P. C. Barton (1786-1856), later a distinguished physician botanist, wrote his University of Pennsylvania thesis, *A Dissertation on the Chymical Properties and Exhilerating Effects of Nitrous-Oxide Gas* (Philadelphia, 1808, 95 pp.). Here was emphasized the brain disorientation caused by inhaling nitrous oxide; we would now call it a psychodelic effect. Barton quoted Davy's words. This report may have inspired itinerant medicine show performers to put on an act demonstrating the effects of inhaling nitrous oxide.

Meanwhile an anonymous note, often ascribed to Michael Faraday, indicated that inhalation of ether would give effects similar to those of nitrous oxide (*Q J Sci, 4*:158-159, 1818). The sweet oil of vitriol, prepared by Valerius Cordus about 1540, was described by J.A.S. Frobensius (d. 1741), who named it ether (*Philos Trans R Soc Lond, 36*:283, 1739). About 1743, the Manchester surgeon, M. Turner, published *An Account of the Extraordinary Medical Fluid Called Aether* (London, n.d.), in which he recommended ether inhalation to relieve pain. The idea was in the air.

Then Henry Hill Hickman (1800-1830) of Britain deliberately experimented with administration of carbon dioxide to dogs to produce surgical anesthesia. His *Letter on Suspended Animation* (Ironbridge, 1824) records his success. Yet he failed to arouse interest and killed himself in frustration. Over a century later Ralph Waters and I, at the University of Wisconsin, confirmed Hickman's findings with the result that about 230 mm Hg carbon dioxide tension with about 530 mm Hg oxygen is used for inhalation therapy in schizophrenia (*Anesth Analg, 8*:17-19, 1929; *Calif West Med, 31*:27-30, 1929).

Then in 1839, William E. Clarke (1818-1878) in Rochester, New York, began the fad of ether frolics among young people. He is alleged to have given ether for extraction of a tooth in 1842. Ether frolics were popular all over the United States. In Jefferson, Georgia, Crawford W. Long (1815-1878) noted that one of the participants in an ether frolic fell heavily but with no indication of pain. On March 30, 1842, he gave ether by inhalation to a patient for removal of a neck tumor with no evidence of pain. The extant bill shows "Operation $2.00; ether 25¢" (Frances Long Taylor, *Crawford W. Long and the Discovery of Ether Anesthesia,* New York City, Hoeber, 1928). Long had been cautioned as a student at the University of Pennsylvania not to burden the medical journals with trivial reports. He failed to report his anesthetic success.

Itinerant medicine shows with demonstration of nitrous oxide effects were also popular. In Hartford, Connecticut, late in 1844, the young dentist, Horace Wells (1815-1848) watched such a nitrous oxide show staged by Gardner Q. Colton (1814-1898). The subject fell but seemed to suffer no pain. Promptly Wells had Colton administer the gas while a colleague pulled a sore tooth. There was no pain. Through his pupil the former partner, William T. G. Morton (1819-1868), a student at Harvard Medical School, Wells arranged to give a demonstration before the surgery class of John Collins Warren (1778-1856) in the Massachusetts General Hospital. The demonstration was a failure, as the patient screamed and struggled. Wells was jeered as "humbug" and retired disgraced.

Morton, who witnessed the fiasco, conferred with Wells and nitrous oxide was used successfully for dental extraction. Morton, however, was not satisfied and sought a more powerful agent. From the erratic Charles T. Jackson (1805-1880) Morton learned of sulfuric ether. Experimenting with this at his home, with various small animals, Morton learned how to administer the volatile substance. He tried to perfect an inhaling device. Again, a demonstration was arranged. The amphitheater on the top floor of the Massachusetts General Hospital was crowded with students eager to scoff again. To quote from my Letheon:

> But Morton failed to come at ten o'clock,
> the appointed time.
> "As Doctor Morton has not yet arrived,"
> said Collins Warren,
> "I presume that he is otherwise engaged."
> Just as raucous laughter followed Warren's jibe,
> Young Morton entered out of breath
> from rushing up the several stairs,
> the new inhaler in his hands . . .
> Then Warren said, "Well, sir, your patient's ready."
>
> . . . So Morton held the inhaler close to (the patient's) mouth
> for many tense and quiet minutes,
> until he seemed to be asleep.
> Then Morton said to Warren,
> "Sir, your patient is prepared."
> As Warren slashed with dextrous hand
> into the tumor, silence startled all.
> There were no shrieks, no violent strife,
> as usually occurred.
> There was merely gentle breathing,
> as in a peaceful sleep.
> In awe they watched the Death of Pain,
> and were convinced.
> Said Warren, "Gentlemen, this is no humbug!"

It is not appropriate here to detail the unpleasant bickering and jockeying which ensued between Wells, Jackson and Morton, as each strove for monetary and prestige reward. The controversy flared in the Congress of the United States, as well as in clinical and scientific circles abroad. All three tried personally to press their claims in France. Much of this discussion calmed when Crawford Long finally published a report on his prior use of ether (*South Med J* n.s. *5:*705-713, 1849).

Actually, the definitive account of the Morton demonstration of ether anesthesia on October 16, 1846 was made by Henry Jacob Bigelow (1818-1890) in an article which attracted world-wide attention (*Bost Med Surg J, 35:*309-317, Nov. 18, 1846). In this ether is compared with nitrous oxide, ethyl nitrate, and alcohol, and it is noted that Morton had already used ether in "upwards of two hundred patients." Vomiting was observed in children, and failure in robust men.

Much experimentation on anesthesia quickly was undertaken. Oliver Wendell Holmes, writing to Morton on November 21, 1846, had proposed the term anesthesia for the condition induced by ether. This word had already been used by Dioscorides to indicate insensibility to pain. In April, 1847, Nikolai Ivanovich Pirigoff (1810-1881), the great Russian surgeon, reported on the rectal administration of ether in oil for anesthesia. Pierre J. M. Flourens (1794-1867), a pupil of Magendie who first analyzed the sense of equilibrium, differentiated etherization from asphyxiation, analyzed the action of ether on the central nervous system, and noted the anesthetic action of chloroform and ethyl chloride in animals (*Comp Rend Acad Sci, 24:*457, 1847).

Chloroform had been independently and simultaneously prepared in 1831 by Samuel Guthrie (1782-1848) of Sacketts Harbor, New York; Eugéne Souberain (1797-1858) of Paris, and Justus Von Liebig (1803-1873) of Darmstadt. Guthrie may also have made ethyl chloride (chloric ether), and Liebig first synthesized chloral. No clinical studies were made on chloroform until James Young Simpson (1811-1870), the great Edinburgh obstetrician, experimented with it in 1847. Simpson was dissatisfied with ether as an agent to relieve delivery pains; it acted too slowly.

From his competent Liverpool friend chemist James Waldie (1813-1889), Simpson received samples of various volatile liquids, including chloric ether, a solution of chloroform in alcohol, and chloroform itself. These were studied by Simpson, using his friends and relatives as subjects, all seated around the big oval table on the ground floor front dining room at 52 Queens Street in Edinburgh. Part of a rest-house for the Church of Scotland, Simpson's bottled samples are still on the shelves in the corner cupboard.

The prompt and powerful action of chloroform immediately impressed Simpson and soon he was using it effectively to relieve pain at childbirth (*Account of a New Anesthetic Agent as a Substitute for Sulphuric Ether,* Edinburgh, 1847, 23 pp.) Simpson's reports were quickly confirmed but there came the usual carping criticisms. One, on religious grounds, castigated Simpson for interfering with the divine curse on women, probably patriarchically inspired, that child-bearing would be accompanied by pain and sorrow. Simpson won the point by the ridiculous argument that anesthesia was divinely authorized when Adam was put to sleep before Eve was born from him. In spite of the vigorous rationality of the mid-nineteenth century, fundamentalism was still supreme. Simpson, however, by his continued publishing on the merits of chloroform, won his point.

The introduction of chloroform anesthesia promoted much debate on the relative merits of ether and chloroform for surgical anesthesia. Opinion divided along national lines: U.S.A. favoring ether, Britain chloroform, and this preferential bias continued for decades. Thomas Nunnely (1809-1870) of Leeds began to study halogenated hydrocarbons and experimented with mixtures of alcohol, chloroform and ether for inhalation anesthesia. The ACE mixture was soon used clinically (*Edin Med Surg J,* 72:357, 1848). Nunnely studied benzene, bromoform, carbon dioxide, carbon disulfide, ethyl bromide, ethyl chloride, ethylene, and methane (*On Anesthesia and Anesthetic Substances Generally: An Experimental Inquiry,* Worcester, 1849, 215 pp.). This was the pioneering comparative pharmacological study of potential inhalation anesthetics from the standpoint of relative effectiveness and safety.

A careful analysis of the clinical aspects of inhalation anesthetics was made by John Snow (1813-1858), the careful Londoner who helped to control cholera by hygienic measures. Snow made quantitative estimates of ether and chloroform concentrations in relation to effects produced, and made inhalation devices. He also studied sudden death during chloroform administration (*On Chloroform And Other Anesthetics: Their Action and Administration,* London, 1858, 443 pp.). Further developments in the pharmacology of anesthetics came in the latter half of the nineteenth century.

Meanwhile remarkable self-experimentation with drugs was by Jan Evangesta Purkyné (1787-1886), the brilliant Czech microscopist and physiologist, whose laboratory in Breslau in 1842 was the first student-teaching workshop in physiology in mid-Europe. Purkyné was a warm humanist and poet, interested in brain activity. It was in the charming baroque of Charles University in Prague that Purkyné, he of the cardiac fibers and the cerebellar cells, did so much of his pharmacological work.

Stimulated by Johann Wolfang von Goethe (1749-1843), Purkyné studied subjective aspects of bodily activity, especially vision. Using ipecac, he well described the nausea produced by it, and then reported in a detailed manner on the effects on vision of belladonna and digitalis (*Beob Vers Physiol d Sinne,* 2:120-128, 1925). He used large doses and had considerable visual disturbance, including flickering, therefrom. He studied the central stimulant action of camphor (trimethyl-bicyclo-2-heptanone), the gum crystals from *Laurus camphora,* the camphor tree of China, Japan and Sumatra, long used natively as a local analgesic and respiratory stimulant. The brain depressant action of opium was studied by him. His were among the most careful studies on ciliary motion, and he noted the effects thereon of several drugs, both from central and local action.

German pharmacology began in the first half of the nineteenth century with Rudolf Buchheim (1820-1879). A pupil of the physiologist E. H. Weber (1795-1878) at Leipzig, Buchheim established his reputation by a German translation, with his own revisions of the comprehensive *Elements of Materia Medica and Therapeutics,* of the London apothecary, Jonathan Pereira (1804-1853). Buchheim eliminated many time-worn folk-remedies, and introduced new discussions on the nature of the effects of drugs

(*Jonathan Pereiras Handbuch der Heilmittellehre*, Leipzig, 2 Vols. 1846, 1848). He then became professor of materia medica in the University of Dorpat, in Esthonia. Here he taught pharmacology on an experimental basis in his own home, reporting on the absorption and excretion of salts of sodium, potassium and calcium, on the action of salts of heavy metals, on the action of alcohol and chloroform, and on anthelmintics and cathartics. Buchheim seems to have been inspired by Magendie's publications. His text, *Lehrbuch der Arzneimittellehre* (Leipzig, 1849), classified drugs on the basis of their main action on various organs of the mammalian body, thus following the organological arrangement of biological information introduced by Albrecht von Haller (1708-1777) in his great nine volume *Elementa physiologiae corporis humani* (Lausanne, 1759-1766). This organ and tissue orientation of physiology and pharmacology is just about yielding now to the broad sweep of the organizational levels of living material from molecules to ecologies. The pupils of Buchheim developed pharmacology in the Germanic areas.

A characteristic feature of the pharmacology of the first half of the nineteenth century was the establishment of toxicology on a firm quantitative base. This began with the Spanish chemist, Mathien Joseph Bonaventura Orfila (1787-1853). From Barcelona, where he received his doctorate in medicine, he went to Paris, where he became professor of legal medicine. Experimenting with arsenical salts in dogs, he noted variation in toxicity under varying conditions and was struck by the lack of quantitative toxicological data. After working with and sacrificing several thousand dogs, he published his famed *Traité des poisons* (2 Vols., Paris, 1814-1815). He demonstrated the value of chemical analysis for evidence of poisoning. For antidotes for poisons taken by mouth, he recommended egg-white, milk, and marshmallow, or gall-nuts and magnesia.

One of Orfila's pupils was the famed Edinburgh medical teacher, Robert Christison (1797-1882). His *Treatise on Poisons* (Edinburgh, 1829) went into several editions. His studies included pioneering investigations of the toxicity of oxalic acid, opium, arsenic and lead salts. He showed that the actions of hemlock and its chief alkaloid, coniine, are practically the same, and the counterpart on the spinal cord, of nux vomica and its alkaloid, strychnine. Particularly striking were his self-experiments with the calabar ordeal bean of West Africa, the seeds of *Physostigma venenosum*. He noted its stimulation of peristalsis and of nausea (*Month J Med Sci, 20:*193-204, 1855).

The Edinburgh tradition of leadership in toxicology was well established in the second half of the nineteenth century. Meanwhile, this tradition was being fostered by the world-wide success of a relatively simple test for the presence of arsenic in body tissues or fluids. This resulted from the work of James Marsh (1794-1846), in which he showed how one might readily separate "small quantities of arsenic from substances with which it may be mixed" (*Edin New Phil J, 21:*229-236, 1836).

Thus it is clear that modern pharmacology rose during the first half of the nineteenth century with the coming of precise methods of chemical analysis. This permitted the isolation of the major alkaloids from various crude drug preparations, some of which had been used from antiquity. With Magendie's genius, quantitative studies of the effects of pure chemicals on living material could be undertaken, and the basic scientific problems of pharmacology could be outlined. The tremendous practical achievement of anesthesia led to systematic investigations of drug actions in depressing pain. German pharmacology made its faltering start, and toxicology was put on a quantitative foundation. Pharmacology as a scientific discipline was being accepted and the ancient descriptive materia medica was being abandoned. The second half of the nineteenth century was to witness many great pharmacological advances, all of which would follow along the paths so well marked by Magendie and his pupils, Bernard and Blake.

CHAPTER 10

PHARMACOLOGY IN THE SECOND HALF OF THE NINETEENTH CENTURY

> Even nectar is poison if taken to excess.
>
> Hindu proverb.

IT IS RATHER FOOLISH to be arbitrary about broad periods of time: the second half of the nineteenth century of our reckoning is really quite continuous with half centuries before and after. Yet, in considering the events comprising the steady increase of verifiable knowledge about the interactions between the molecules of drugs and living material—the growth of pharmacology—it is convenient to relate those events to the general milieu of their time. Thus, we do make convenient groupings of time in order to relate to one another rather than to run along in the continuum that really is the case. It is so easy to get lost by following one path alone.

Characteristic of pharmacology in the first half of the nineteenth century was the isolation in chemically pure form of the biologically active agents of crude drugs used empirically for ages. With pure chemicals of constant physico chemical properties, one could begin quantitative studies on the varying biological responses to varying dosage. Physicians, dentists and veterinarians could have confidence in the probable response of their patients to the same dose of a uniform pure drug. This resulted in careful appraisal of effectiveness and toxicity on single and repeated administration. The desire then arose to find, or to create, substitutes for the natural products in order to reduce costs, as in the case of quinine, or to get greater effectiveness with less toxicity, as in the case of inhalation anesthetics.

Thus the search for new and better drugs began. Characteristic of the pharmacology of the second half of the nineteenth century was the remarkable and often serendipitous success attendant upon this search. It was the rise of chemistry that made this possible. Qualitative and quantitative chemical analysis became well standardized and reliable. The atomic theory of John Dalton (1766-1844) made it possible readily to understand the composition of inorganic compounds. The dreamily imaginative Friedrich August Kekulé von Stradonitz (1829-1896) of Darmstadt provided the clue to an understanding of the composition of aromatic organic compounds. With the discovery of various methods of chemical synthesis, the way was open to the deliberate effort to find synthetic substitutes for the biologically active compounds from natural sources. Impetus to this effort came from economic pressure (as in the increasing cost of quinine from the depleted cinchona forests of Peru), or from clinical pressure to get drugs which would be more effective and safer for specific purposes than any available. These factors continue to operate, now, unfortunately, enmeshed with political, legal and bureaucratic ineptness.

If, as James Blake surmised and found, there is a relationship between the chemical constitution of a drug and its biological activity, then knowledge of the physiochemical makeup of a drug should aid in giving a clue to the physicochemical structure of the molecules of living materials with which the molecules of that drug would interact. Blake implied the concept of the target locus of action in living material in the first half of the nineteenth century. Neglect of Blake's idea delayed the development of what is now called "molecular pharmacology" until the present time. This is comparable to the long neglect of the potential value of nitrous-oxide and ether for effective anesthesia.

The pharmacology and toxicology of anesthetic agents was widely explored in the latter half of our nineteenth century. Successful local anesthesia was achieved and well developed. By 1853, Edward R. Squibb (1819-1900) had devised a method for the large scale production of relatively pure ether for anesthesia, blowing a hand off in the process. This opened the way for the industrial production of standardized drugs, and the now huge drug industry was on the way.

Although the principle of a tube and syringe for administering drugs had long been known, as in the clyster for enemas or even for intravenous injection, it was not until 1853 that the hypodermic needle and syringe as we know it, was first used. Alexander Wood (1817-1884) devised it for the parenteral administration of drugs in solution, the instrument being convenient for cleaning *(Edin Med Surg J, 82:265-281, 1853)*. He used it to apply morphine directly to painful joints.

It was on April 7, 1853 that Queen Victoria submitted to the use of Simpson's chloroform at the delivery of her eighth child, Prince Leopold. John Snow was the anesthetist. This even silenced social and religious opposition to the use of anesthetics in obstetrics. At the London International Exhibition in 1862, Joseph Thomas Clover (1825-1882) showed an apparatus "to regulate with precision the mixture of air and chloroform vapor, and to limit the proportion of the latter to four and a half in a hundred." Chloroform, being neither explosive nor flammable, had a marked advantage over ether, but it was more powerful and potentially more toxic. Clover was wise in trying to limit the concentration to be used.

In 1863 Gardner Quincy Colton (1814-1898), who first gave nitrous-oxide for anesthetic purposes to Horace Wells in 1844, now successfully revived its use in dentistry for pulling teeth. Five years later in Paris, he demonstrated nitrous-oxide for dental anesthesia. This stimulated Clover to adapt his chloroform inhaler to nitrous oxide. Alfred Coleman (1828-1902) became the chief exponent of the use of nitrous-oxide in dentistry and introduced a carbondioxide absorber as an economizer. English manufacturers successfully compressed nitrous-oxide into metal cylinders with delivery valves, thus greatly facilitating its use. It was still thought that nitrous-oxide acted in part by asphyxiation. Edmund Andrews (1824-1904) successfully overcome this objection by administering nitrous-oxide with oxygen *(Chicago Med Exam, 9:656-661, 1868)*.

Meanwhile, unexplained deaths with chloroform led to the selection of a Chloroform Commission by the Royal Medical and Chirurgical Society to study the problem. The committee report *(Med Chir Trans, 47:323-442, 1864)* recognized the greater safety of ether. It was gradually realized that vagal stimulation as a result of local laryngeal irritation on first inhaling chloroform might be enough to stop the heart. J. A. F. Dastre (1844-1917) of Paris recommended pre-medication with atropine to prevent vagal stoppage of the heart *(Compt Rend Acad Sci, 86*:1303, 1878). Difficulties with chloroform continued and resulted in the Nizam of Hyderabad giving funds for two consecutive committees to study the problem. The reports were inconclusive and excited much discussion. It was gradually recognized that prolonged or frequently repeated administrations of chloroform would injure the liver. Hepatotoxicity is characteristic of halogenated hydrocarbon anesthetic agents. It has also been found that chloroform anesthesia is prone to result in sudden blocking of normal cortical inhibitory impulses, thus bringing epinephrine release from the adrenal glands with resulting cardiovascular syncope (A. G. Levy, *Chloroform Anesthesia,* London, 1922, 166 pp). The long effort to understand the difficulties of chloroform anesthesia resulted in much pharmacological impetus, and in clarifying many details of the various mechanisms of drug action.

Meanwhile, Benjamin Ward Richardson (1828-1896), pupil and biographer of John Snow, used a hand bellows to spray a cloud of ether on the skin, where rapid evaporation would produce cold sufficient to give short local anesthesia, enough to permit opening a superficial abscess without pain. Later ethyl chloride was used for this purpose and still is (P. Redard, *Verh Xth Internat Med Cong, Berlin, 5:*14 Abt., 71-73, 1890).

Richardson, the genial medical biographer and temperance advocate, undertook a systematic pharmacological study of alcohols, hydrocarbons, and halogenated hydrocarbons. He noted that there is quantitative increase in single dose toxicity with increase in number of carbon atoms in straight-carbon-chained alcohols, until there is a qualitative change in physicochemical properties. "Richardson's principle" has been widely applied in the synthesis of many alkyl compounds for drug use, as exemplified in the important *Arzneimittelsynthese* (Springer, Berlin, 1901) of Sigmund Fränkel (1868-1942?). An excellent analysis of Richardson's contribution to the rise of molecular pharmacology, as well as Blake's pioneering effort, was made by William F. Bynum *(Bull Hist Med, 44:*518-538, 1970). Bynum well discusses the fascinating history of biochemorphology.

Richardson also showed the vasodilating action of amyl nitrite on inhalation. This compound had been made by Antoine Jerome Balard (1802-1876) of Paris *(Comp Rend Acad Sci, 19:*634-641, 1859). Arthur Gamgee (1841-1909) demonstrated its blood-pressure lowering action to the Scotsman, Thomas Lauder Brunton (1844-1916), who tried it for relief of angina pectoris with prompt success *(Lancet, 2:*97-98, 1867). Subsequently, many organic nitrates were devised for prolonging the relief from anginal pain.

Nitroglycerine, either triturated to 1 percent with lactose in small tablets or in 1 percent solution in alcohol (spirits of glyonin), was introduced as a longer acting vasodilator than amyl nitrite by William Murrell (1853-1912), and it is still the generally used drug for relief of acute angina pectoris *(Lancet, 1:*80, 113, 151, 225, 1879). Erythrol-tetranitrate and other similar organic nitrates are also widely used. The biochemorphology of the organic nitrates was well analyzed *(Philos Trans R Soc Lond, 184:*505-639, 1894) by John Theodore Cash (1854-1936) and Wyndham Rowland Dunstan (1861-1949). More recently the pharmacology of the nitrates has been examined by John Christian Krantz, Jr. (1899-   ), and by Lathan Crandall and myself.

Lauder Brunton also studied the cardiac strengthening effect of digitalis in relation to its diuretic action. He investigated the diuretic effect of the well-known purgative, calomel (mercurous chloride), and of other nontoxic mercury compounds.

Brunton, a pupil of Carl Ludwig (1816-1895) the great Berlin physiologist, established a pioneer teaching laboratory for pharmacology in a tiny scullery in St. Bartholomew's Hospital, London, in which he actually paid students to work for him! His *Text Book of Pharmacology, Therapeutic and Materia Medica* (London, 1885) became a popular and widely-used reference source for drug use. This contained much inspiration for the study of the relationship between the chemical constitution of organic compounds and their biological action. No mention was made of Blake's earlier work on this matter with respect to inorganic salts. In Blake's copy of Brunton's text, Blake had written "bosh" in the page margin where Brunton started his discussion of the subject!

At Edinburgh, Brunton was acquainted with Thomas Richard Fraser (1841-1920), who had continued Christison's study of the calabar bean, extracting the alkaloid physostigmine from it. This, he found, constricts the pupil, slows the heart, promotes lachrymal and salivary secretion, and increases intestinal activity.

Further, he showed that atropine prevents or reverses these effects, thus demonstrating a basic antagonism between the actions of atropine and physostigmine. This observation helped later in the analysis of the balanced and reciprocal physiological activity of the autonomic nervous system in regard to its thoracolumbar (or sympathetic) and its craniosacral (or parasympathetic) components.

Fraser became Christison's assistant and succeeded him as Professor of Materia Medicia in 1877. With his chemist colleague, Alexander Crum Brown (1838-1922), Fraser made an important observation relating the chemical makeup of various alkaloids to their biological activity. They showed, with strychnine, brucine, thebaine, codeine, morphine and nicotine, that changing the nitrogen in the compound from a tertiary form to a quaternary ammonium base resulted in a chemical agent with uniform curare-like activity in mammals, regardless of its original characteristic biological effect. Thus, whereas these alkaloids have a generally convulsive effect in high dose, they become less toxic as the quaternary compound and show a general muscular paralyzing action. With atropine and coniine, however, this structural change results in greater toxicity. This finding ("On the connection between chemical constitution and physiological action," *Trans R Soc Edin, 25:* 151-203, 1868-69) is frequently said to have been the first investigation of the relationship between the chemical structure and biological action (biochemorphology), but actually it was anticipated by twenty years by James Blake in regard to inorganic salts.

Fraser also carefully studied the African arrow poison strophanthus ("Strophanthus hispidus: its natural history, chemistry and pharmacology," *Trans R Soc Edin, 35:*955-1027, 1890; *36:*343-457, 1892), and introduced standardized preparations of it for rapid strengthening of failing hearts. His versatility as a brilliant pharmacologist was further shown in his studies on cobra venom and on methods of immunization against its action by means of an antivenom serum *(Br Med J, 1*:1309-1312, 1895). Similar findings were reported in Paris by Albert Léon Charles Calmette (1863-1933). The latter's studies included several types of venoms and were brought together in book form *(Le vénin des serpents,* Paris, 1896). My special study of the development of knowledge about venoms recently appeared *(Venomous Animals and Their Venoms,* Eds.: W. Bucherl, Eleanor Buckley and V. Deulofen, New York, Academic Press, 1968, pp. 1-12).

When I visited the Pharmacology Laboratory of the University of Edinburgh in 1938, the distinguished Professor of Materia Medica, Alfred Joseph Clark (1885-1941), proudly showed me the various crude drug specimens so painstakingly gathered by Fraser, together with the original samples of the active agents isolated from them, and the original records of experiments on them. This material was well displayed in a useful teaching cabinet. Later I was told that after Clark's death, this precious exhibit was thrown away. This so discouraged me that when I was in Edinburgh a few years ago, I could not get myself to go to the Laboratory for fear it might be true!

The Rise of German Pharmacology

Rudolf Buchheim (1820-1879) is generally recognized as the conceptual pioneer for German pharmacology. Deprecating both pharmacy and chemistry, he emphasized the necessity of investigating drug action in a systematic way in order to give a rational background for drug therapy. He was influential in turning attention from the identification and standardization of drugs (materia medica) to the scientific study of their interactions with living material, which is pharmacology *(Beiträge zur Arzneimittellehre,* Leipzig, 1849). He was a keen teacher at Dorpat, and his most famous pupil was Oswald Schmiedeberg (1838-1921) who succeeded him in 1866.

France was greatly humiliated in the Franco-Prussian War, and its scientific prestige faltered. Alsace-Lorraine was Prussianized and the victors sought to make an intellectual show-place of Strassburg. Many young German scientists were brought there, among them Schmiedeberg. The University was refurbished and expanded. For Schmiedeberg, who came to Strassburg in 1872, a new and well-equipped pharmacology institute was built. The first of its kind anywhere, it soon attracted a flock of over one hundred students from twenty countries! Ambitious American youngsters deserted Paris for Germany, and those interested in the new and formally recognized science of pharmacology went to Strassburg to become devoted pupils of Schmiedeberg. The excellence of his teaching justified their expectations.

Schmiedeberg, while at Dorpat with his pupil, Richard Koppec, wrote a classic report *Das Muscarin: Das Giftige Alkaloid des Fliegenpilzes* (Leipzig, Vogel, 1869). In this, they were the first to show the similarity between the effect of a drug and the effect of electrical stimulation by demonstrating that muscarine and electrical stimulation of the vagus nerves slow heart movement, and that both are antagonized by atropine. The muscarine and vagal stimulation effects were shown to be localized at the nerve endings and not in heart muscle. They described the isolation of the alkaloid, its physicochemical properties, its biological activity, and its toxicity in relation to mushroom poisoning from *Amanita muscaria* from which it is obtained.

Schmiedeberg was influential in directing attention to mechanisms of drug detoxification and drug removal from living material. W. Keller had shown that ingested benzoic acid is excreted as hippuric acid *(Ann Chem Pharm, 43:*108-111, 1842). Schmiedeberg realized that the appearance of hippuric acid in the urine after ingestion of benzoic acid was due to simple conjugation of the latter with glycine, an amino acid naturally occurring in the body. He showed that conjugation occurs in the kidney rather than in the liver and that the resulting hippuric acid is rapidly excreted into the urine. His experiment with George Bunge (1844-1920) including perfusion of isolated kidneys *(Arch Exp Pathol Pharmakol, 6:*233-255, 1875). It was realized that this perfusion technique would help in the study of many problems involving vertebrate metabolism. It also pointed the way to kidney dialysis.

By similar experimental studies, Schmiedeberg showed that

urea is formed in the liver, and that organic drug components may conjugate with glucuronic acid to be excreted in the urine. He initiated studies on the chemistry and detailed activity of digitalis preparations, recognizing the character of the digitalis glucosides *(Arch Exp Pathol Pharmakol, 16:*149-187, 1883). So many were the findings of his students in his new Strassburg laboratory, that in 1873 he established and edited *Archives für Experimentelle Pathologie und Pharmakologie,* generally known as *Schmiedeberg's Archives.* This was very important in establishing the prestige of pharmacology as an independent scientific discipline. Similarly, his text, *Grundriss der Arzneimittellehre* (Leipzig, Vogel, 1883), aided greatly in promoting the importance of pharmacology in medical training and practice.

Schmiedeberg's successor at Dorpat was Rudolf Böhm (1844-1926), who had been a pupil of the famed physiologist Carl Ludwig (1816-1895) at Leipzig. In 1889 Böhm became Professor of Pharmacology at Leipzig. He isolated and characterized the active anthelmintic agents in the anciently used male fern *(Dryopteris filix-mas),* and of such cathartics as *Cascara sagrada* and croton oil. He recognized that the pure active agents, such as emodin, are too irritating for practical use, and that the crude drugs are safer and preferable, since the tannins and gums in them reduce the local irritation of the active ingredients. He noted disappearance of liver glycogen in chloroform anesthesia, and studied the effects of various chemical modifications such as methylation on alkaloidal activity. Without reference to James Blake, he studied the antagonistic action of potassium and calcium salts on isolated or perfused hearts. He noted the cardiac effects of barium salts and investigated acute poisoning with arsenic, antimony, and platinum salts and also with elementary phosphorus.

A famed pupil of Schmiedeberg's, Hans Horst Meyer (1853-1939), succeeded Böhm at Dorpat in 1881 and again at Marburg in 1884. In 1904 he became Professor of Pharmacology at Vienna; he would later develop a renowned Institute there. With Schmiedeberg he had discovered the detoxifying action of glucuronic acid, and with Emil Adolf Von Behring (1854-1917), he studied tetanus toxin. He showed that the toxin is absorbed by peripheral nerves and carried in their axons to the central nervous system and brain. Meyer demonstrated that calcium ions decrease capillary and lymph vessel permeability.

Von Behring helped to develop Japanese pharmacology by his brilliant work with Shibasaburo Kitasato (1852-1931) in discovering and standardizing diphtheria and tetanus antioxins *(Deutsche Med Wochenschr, 16:*1113-1114, 1890). The standardization was affected by adjusting products to the biological strength of an arbitrary preparation and expressing dosage in terms of units of the standard. This became the usual methodology for immune preparations, and later for vitamins, hormones and many crude drugs. Von Behring was awarded the first Nobel prize in medicine in 1900.

Hans Horst Meyer is well known for his theory of narcosis *(Arch Exp Pathol Pharmakol, 42:*109-118, 1899). His analysis of hydrocarbon, alcohol and anesthetic narcosis is masterful and proceeds from Schmiedeberg's dictum that the hydrocarbon groups of aliphatic substances are responsible for their narcotic effect. The conclusion he reached is that the relative strength of narcotic drugs depends on their relative affinities for fats and for water, a relation expressed by a partition coefficient. The greater the solubility of a compound in lipid material in comparison with its solubility in water, the greater its narcotizing power. Actually this is more of a theory explaining the distribution of anesthetic agents in living material (nerves are rich in lipids) than an explanation of the mechanism of anesthesia. Yet it has been very influential in the study of anesthetic agents.

Meyer's theory received prompt support from the more detailed analyses of the Englishman Charles Ernest Overton (1865-1933). After long service in Zürich and Würzburg, Overton became Professor of Pharmacology at Lund in 1907. As a botanist, Overton was interested in the permeability of cells for various substances. He noted that narcosis in tadpoles occurred when certain amounts of simple aliphatic compounds penetrated the cells he was studying. This led him to investigate narcosis in relation to the chemical constitution of aliphatic compounds, beginning with alcohols *(Studien über die Narkose,* Jean, 1910). Like Richardson, Overton observed greater potency with an increase in the length of a carbon chain up to an optimum. He also noted decrease in activity when a hydrogen or halogen atom is replaced by hydroxyl. He concluded that the narcotic strength of a substance is determined by its partition coefficient between watery and lecithin-cholesterol-like solvents in cells. Overton's detailed analysis resulted in calling the oil-water partition coefficient theory of anesthesia, the Meyer-Overton Theory.

It was not, however, adequate to explain the mechanism of anesthesia. Thomas Butler, in reviewing various theories of anesthesia, concluded that none was satisfactory *(Pharmacol Rev, 2:*121-160, 1950). The more recent clathrate crystal theory of anesthesia, proposed by Linus Pauling *(Science, 134:*15-21, 1961), was extended to an "ice-cover" theory by S. L. Miller *(Proc Natl Acad Sci, 47:*1515-1524, 1961). Robert Featherstone and C. A. Muehlbacher further cast doubt on the basic significance of the Meyer-Overton lipid-water solubility anesthesia theory by indicating that proteins have greater importance in anesthesia than lipids, thus returning to Claude Bernard's proposals of a century earlier *(Pharmacol Rev, 15:*97-121, 1963). Leroy D. Vandam has well reviewed the current scientific status of anesthesia *(Ann Rev Pharmacol, 6:*379-414, 1966).

Meanwhile, successful local anesthesia for surgical and dental anesthesia was achieved, thanks to the discernment of Carl Koller (1857-1944). Koller was an intern in the Allgemeine Krankenhaus in Vienna working with his friend, Sigmund Freud (1856-1939). Freud had a distinguished patient who had become addicted to morphine, a characteristic central nervous depressant. Freud thought the addiction to morphine might be counteracted by a central nervous system stimulant. The central stimulating effect of cocaine had been noted, but in 1884 it was still something of a chemical curiosity. Freud had himself published a brief monograph on cocaine, without, however, arousing much interest. Among other proposed uses for cocaine, Freud suggested it as a means of controlling alcohol or morphine addiction.

Vasili K. Anrep (1852-   ) had noted the numbing action of cocaine on the tongue when the alkaloid was tasted, and recognized that this numbing effect was a manifestation of local anesthesia

(Arch Ges Physiol, 21:38-77, 1880). Others had also commented on this action of cocaine. Freud proposed a careful study of cocaine and enlisted the interest of his colleague, Carl Koller. While Freud was on a visit to his fiancée, Carl continued the study.

Koller, however, had determined to become an ophthalmologist, and was anxious to find something which could be placed directly in an eye to anesthetize it for a cataract operation without having the inconvenience of an inhaler or towel over the face for general anesthesia.

Koller himself relates how the idea of using cocaine as a local anesthetic for the eyes suddenly struck him one day in the laboratory. He promptly made experiments on the eyes of guinea-pigs, rabbits and dogs, and convinced that cocaine solution could indeed anesthetize the eyes, confirmed such action on his own eyes and on those of his colleagues.

Koller's publication *(Wien Med Wchnschr, 34*:1276-1278, 1309-1311, 1884) is a model of detailed pharmacological reporting with special emphasis on practical applications in eye surgery. His findings had been demonstrated for him at the Heidelberg Opthalmological Congress on September 15, 1884. Koller himself could not afford to attend. The significance of his discovery was promptly appreciated; his work, in translation and in editorial comment, appeared in many medical journals. Freud gallantly disclaimed any credit for the discovery, and Koller himself took pains in a letter to the editor of the *Vienna Journal,* dated December 17, 1884, to refer to Anrep's previous studies as well as to those of others. Properly he deserves full credit for introducing cocaine local anesthesia for eye surgery. Very quickly cocaine was used for infiltration local anesthesia and even spinal anesthesia in general surgery.

Koller, unfortunately, in resenting an insult from a colleague early in 1885, was challenged to a duel, in which he was the victor. His position in Vienna became precarious, and he fortunately secured a place with Franciscus Cornelis Donders (1818-1889) at the Nederlandsche Gasthuis voor Ooglijders in Utrecht. Here he completed his opthalmological training and in 1889 migrated to New York City. Throughout his difficulties, Freud remained his encouraging friend. The full story, with many quotations from letters, is given in the account by his daughter, Mrs. Hortense Koller (James H.) Becker of Highland Park, Illinois *(Psychoanal Q, :32* 309-373, 1963).

Here I may be pardoned for inserting a personal note. As a boy I lived in Elizabeth, New Jersey, and when I was about ten years old, I had difficulty reading. A young eye specialist told my mother that I was going blind, but that he could prevent it at a cost of ten dollars a week. This was beyond our family budget, so our family physician, Victor Mravlag, who was Mayor of the City, was consulted. He told my mother to take me to an opthalmologist whose office was on Madison Avenue in New York City. The journey was a mere fifteen miles, but in those days with train, ferry and crosstown trolley cars, it was slow and exciting. The reception room in the brownstone house was dignified and quiet. The examination by the awecome doctor in the darkened instrument-filled room was short but frightening. His verdict was that I was astigmatic and nearsighted. The prescription he gave my mother was signed Carl Koller, and the glasses were quickly made by Meyrowitz on Fifth Avenue.

Twenty years later in 1926, when I had learned who Carl Koller was, I returned to his large and handsome office on the second floor of a building on the corner of 59th Street and Madison Avenue. He examined me again and then told me of his work in Vienna and his friendly association with Freud. At my suggestion, he wrote an account of how his discovery was made and exploited *(JAMA, 90:*1742-1743, 1928). In 1934 Carl Koller was made an honorary member of the American Society of Pharmacology and Experimental Therapeutics.

Significant pharmacological developments in local anesthetic agents and their application in practice followed within a couple decades. Before the end of the nineteenth century, Alfred Einhorn had coupled amino-benzoic acid with diethylaminoethanol to form what he called novocaine. *(Münch Med Wchnschr, 46:*1218-1220, 1254-1256, 1899). This was the direct result of the recognition of the potential toxicity of cocaine, especially its addictive properties, and the urge to get a safe and effective local anesthetic agent.

The great Johns Hopkins surgeon, William Stewart Halsted

(1852-1922), had early reported on the use and abuse of cocaine *(N Y Med J, 42:*294-295, 1885), and had himself become addicted to the feeling of exhilaration it gave him after he had accidentally ingested some as he prepared solutions for use. Bravely he learned to control his acquired craving. James Leonard Corning (1855-1923) had introduced spinal anesthesia with cocaine *(N Y Med J, 42:*483-485, 1885), and Carl Ludwig Schleich (1859-1922) had developed infiltration anesthesia *(Ther Monatsh, 8:*429-436, 1894).

The great Munich chemist, Richard Willstätter (1872-1942) was revealing the chemical structure of cocaine and its relation to atropine. This was suggested in 1887 by Wilhelm Filehne (1844-1927) who had introduced antipyrine in 1884 as a quinine substitute. He noted the local anesthetic action of atropine, the active ingredient of belladonna, and surmised that the two similarly acting alkaloids are chemically related. Both have benzoic acid couplings with methyl amino rings. Einhorn reduced the complexity of the natural product to its simplest effective synthetic form.

Procaine (Novocaine) remains the safest local anesthetic for infiltration or spinal anesthesia, but it is not powerful enough to anesthetize an intact mucous membrane. As was shown later by my teacher Arthur S. Loevenhart (1878-1929), the isopropyl diethylamino derivative is strong enough to anesthetize mucous membranes, but is no more toxic than procaine *(J Pharmacol Exp Ther, 24:*159-175, 1924). However, no drug manufacturer was interested in furnishing it, as its sale was not controllable by patent. Some twenty related compounds have since been exploited on the basis of patent rights. Richardson's principle can be noted as operating in them all. At least a dozen other more complex local anesthetic compounds have been derived from Einhorn's pioneering study.

Central Nervous System Depressing and Sleep-producing Drugs

Somewhere at the beginning of the second half of the nineteenth century an idea gained currency that potassium bromide would cause drowsiness. I have not been able to trace the origin of this notion, although I'd like to believe it came from James Blake's work. There is no evidence that this is so. Yet, a report that this inorganic salt causes depression in animals was made by Robert Mortimer Glover (1816-1859) in 1842 *(Edin Med Surg J).* This could be an early reflection of Blake's work. Glover also was the first to report on the use of iodoform as a skin antiseptic *(Edin Month J.* 1847) and on the biological action of picrotoxin, a non-nitrogen active agent from *Anamirta cocculus,* the fish-berry used as a fish poison in the East Indies *(Edin Month J,* 1851).

It was Charles Locock (1799-1875), a popular London obstetrician, who first reported in a professional discussion on the use of potassium bromide in epilepsy *(Lancet, 1:528,* 1857). He had given it for relief of dysmenorrhea and noted a cessation of epileptic seizures in several of his patients after taking the drug.

H. Behrend (of whom I can find little) reported *(Lancet, 1: 607-608,* 1864) that he had used potassium bromide to treat insomnia, nervous excitement and irritability. Reference is made to Alfred Barin Garrod's (1819-1879) lecture comment that potassium bromide causes drowsiness. It is clear that the subject was under discussion. Garrod, who lectured on materia medica, discovered uric acid in the blood of patients with gout and used lithium chloride in its treatment.

The pharmacology of potassium bromide and its success in managing epilepsy were well discussed by Thomas Smith Clouston (1841-1915) of Edinburg *(J Ment Sci, 14:305,* 1868). It was clear that the anticonvulsive action was due to the bromide ion, perhaps by displacement of chloride in nerve cells. Soon the use of triple bromide, i.e. lithium, sodium and potassium bromides, became popular.

A great advance in the rationale of the design of a synthetic drug for a specific purpose was made by the Olympian, Oscar Liebreich (1839-1908). This was the development of chloral hydrate as a sleep-producing agent. *(Das Chloralhydrat: Ein neue Hypnoticum und Anaestheticum,* Berlin, Muller, 1869). Chloral hydrate, $CH(OH)_2$-CCl_3, had been prepared by Liebig in 1862. Liebreich reasoned that in the alkaline reaction of the body, this would slowly be converted to chloroform, $CHCl_3$, and that gentle sleep would result. It can be given by mouth in water solution and is quickly absorbed. Clinically it was successful and promptly filled a great need. Actually, however, it goes to trichlorethanol in the body and as such it is excreted in the urine. It is still widely used, but was once badly abused in *Micky Finns* for dubious purposes. Several related compounds were later developed, including a sugar-chloral combination, chloralose, widely used in England as an anesthetic in experimental animals. Chlorbutanol (Chloretone) was similarly used. In 1871, Liebreich became Professor of Pharmacology at Berlin, and in 1883 in institute was built for him. He developed hydrated wool fat (lanolin) for dermatological use.

Another of Schmiedeberg's famed pupils, Vincenzo Cervello (1854-1919), introduced paraldehyde as an effective and safe soporific *(Arch Ital Biol, 6:*113-114, 1884). Though it often gives an offensive odor and may cause stomach irritation, it was widely used. Meanwhile, the central nervous system depressing effects of ethanol were investigated again by Josef Von Mering (1849-1908). He had shown that chloral hydrate is partly excreted in the urine coupled to glucuronic acid. He found that tertiary alcohols were similarly handled. He noted that secondary alcohols are more depressing than primary and that tertiary ones are still more so. His work led later to the use of amylene hydrate both as a solvent and as an adjuvant for tribromoethanol, to form the potent rectal anesthetic, Avertin. Fritz Eichholtz (1889-1968) introduced this combination into clinical practice *(Deutsch Med Wchnschr, 53:*712-713, 1927).

Von Mering had shown in 1886 the glycosuria resulting from the administration of phloridzin, a glucoside from the root bark of fruit trees. With Oscar Minkowski (1858-1931), he showed that removing the pancreas of dogs would result promptly in the appearance of diabetes mellitus *(Arch Exp Pathol Pharmakol, 26:* 371-387, 1890). This led to the search for the active principle in the pancreas which regulates carbohydrate metabolism in mammals.

Von Mering greatly advanced an understanding of biochemorphology by his studies on the soporific action of alcohols and similar substances. He pointed out that chloral hydrate and its derivatives are related to paraldehyde, a polymeric form of acetaldehyde from which chloral hydrate can be obtained by chlorination. He devised chloralformamide, weaker and safer than chloral hydrates, by applying an idea originating with Schmiedeberg. The latter, noting how ammonia raises blood pressure and stimulates respiration, thought of combining an amino group with a narcotic hydrocarbon, in order to get a soporific without depressant action on circulation or respiration. Carbamic acid, related to urea, was combined with alcohol to form urethane. $NH_2\text{-}CO\text{-}OC_2H_5$. This crystalline compound is a mild narcotic. It had been prepared by Jean Baptiste André Dumas (1800-1884) in 1838. Schmiedeberg recognized it as a compound with the chemical properties he had postulated. Dumas had isolated methyl alcohol in 1834 and had shown its relation to ethanol.

Von Mering was also greatly impressed by the accidental but practical success of the chemist Eugen Baumann (1846-1896) and Alfred Kast (1856-1903) in developing sulphonal, $(CH_3)_2 C(SO_2C_2H_5)_2$, and its ethyl derivatives as efficient and safe soporifics *(Baumann: Ber Deutsch Chem Ges, 19:2806-2814, 1886; Kast: Berl Klin Wchnschr, 25:304-314, 1888)*.

Kast had also introduced the antipyretic analgesic agent, acetophenetidin, in 1887. The German drug makers were now becoming commercially conscious; acetophenetidin was trademarked phenacetin in order to protect its sales.

As Von Mering indicated, the disulfones are somewhat similar to amylene hydrate, and since narcotic action increases with the number of ethyl groups, trional, with three ethyl groups is superior to sulfonal with two. With the aid of Emil Fischer, a biochemist (1852-1919), who was studying purines and uric acid, Von Mering sought a series of compounds similar to the sulphonals but containing a urea moiety. An example is diethyl acetyl urea, $(C_2H_5)_2 CHCONHCONH_2$, which was found to be equal to sulphonal as a soporific. By doubling the urea and closing the ring, Fischer and Von Mering obtained diethyl-malonyl-urea, which actually had been synthesized in 1882 by Conrad Gutzeit. This was found to have a more effective soporific action than diethylacetyl urea, and with a safer, less prolonged response than with dipropylmalonyl urea. Clinical trials were successful. Fischer was in Verona, Italy when Von Mering telegraphed the good news. In honor of the quiet, restful place where the news came, the drug was named Veronal® and thus trademarked.

The report on the new drug *(Ther Gegenw, 44:*97-101, 1903) has been well translated by Holmsted and Liljestrand *(Readings in Pharmacology,* Oxford, 1963, pp. 128-134). In it Fischer and Von Mering referred to several of the obviously many derivatives of barbituric acid or hydropyrimidines which are possible. Over a thousand substitutions of alkyl groups are possible at the C-5 position alone. Many of these have been made patented, trademarked, and exploited. My colleague, Milton Silverman, the keen science writer, has told the story well with imaginative insight, in his *Magic in a Bottle* (New York, Macmillan, 1941. pp. 192-212).

The long, slow acting phenyl-ethyl-malonylurea, trademarked Luminal®, was introduced by Alfred Hauptmann (1881-1948) for the effective and safe treatment of epilepsy *(Munch Med Wchnschr, 59:*1907-1909, 1912).

The value of a perpetual trademark was well illustrated in the case of Veronal and Luminal. So well had these names been publicized that when the patents ran out and the compounds could be competitively made under the public names, barbital and phenobarbital, respectively, the wholesale price of the trademarked preparations could be maintained at relatively high levels. If a physician prescribes a drug under its trademarked name, the pharmacist must supply it as designated. With advertising, trademarked drugs are kept before physicians, and prices are kept high.

In order to bring the story of the increasingly successful treatment of epilepsy up-to-date, it should be noted that Fischer and Von Mering studied hydantoins, including the diethyl compound. The hydantoins are five-membered, double nitrogen-containing rings, instead of the six-membered malonyl urea ring.

Tracy Jackson Putnam (1894-   ) of Harvard became interested in the treatment of epilepsy. With the new electroencephalograph, he could observe the electrical storms in the brain and their subsidence under treatment with phenobarbital. In order to intensify the effect he searched for related chemicals having a diphenyl substituent. From Parke-Davis in Detroit he obtained several compounds, among which was diphenyl hydantoin. This greatly raised the convulsive threshold in experimental cats when a quantitated electrical stimulus was applied to the brain.

With his friend, H. Houston Merritt (1902-   ), Putnam gave diphenylhydantoin to epileptic patients with full success and with few undesired side effects *(Arch Neurol Psychiat, 39:*1003-1015, 1938). The interesting story of the development of Dilantin® therapy of epilepsy has been modestly recounted by Tracy Putnam *(Discoveries in Biological Psychiatry,* Philadelphia, Lippincott, 1971, pp. 85-90).

Antipyretic Analgesics

The increasingly high price of quinine as a result of the reduction of the source of quinine supply with the uncontrolled cutting of the Peruvian cinchona trees stimulated search for effective substitutes for quinine in the management of fevers. It was found that the molecule of quinine contains benzene rings, and quinoline was isolated. This is a double ring system with nitrogen in one of the rings.

Meanwhile aniline had been isolated from coal tar by William Henry Perkin (1838-1907) who developed the great aniline dye industry. Aniline was probably found by accidental contact with it in reducing fever. It is absorbed through the skin. Before this, however, Friedlieb Ferdinand Runge (1795-1867) had prepared carbolic acid, or phenol, from coal tar. Its antiseptic properties were described by François Jules Lemaire (1814-1886) who called it a powerful disinfectant *(Du Coaltar Saporine,* Bailliere, Paris, 1860). Promptly, it was successfully used by Joseph Lister (1827-1912) in surgery to kill bacteria in wounds and to prevent suppuration *(Lancet, 1:*326-329, 1867; *2:*353-356, 1867). This was the practical clinical application of the demonstration of the fermenting and suppurating effects of bacterial action by the brilliant Louis Pasteur (1822-1895). In addition to its antiseptic action, phenol was found to reduce fevers. It is much too toxic, however, as is aniline, to be used for this purpose.

Three decades before, Rafael Piria (1815-1865) had isolated salicin, the active principle of the bark or the leaves of the willow, Salix, decoctions of which were used from antiquity for the relief of the pains and inflammation associated with arthritis and rheumatism. From salicin, salicylic acid was prepared. This is the ortho carboxyl substituted derivative of phenol. It also is mildly antiseptic and antipyretic, but it is too locally irritating to be useful as a medicament by mouth. Its ability painlessly to destroy epithelium is widely used in cornplasters. Willow pastes had been recommended by Dioscorides to treat corns!

The toxicity of aniline, phenol, and salicylic acid was found to be controllable by simple acetylation, combined with acetic acid under proper conditions. I have not been able to trace the sequence of events in the preparation of these acetylated derivatives. Acetylsalicylic acid seems to have been synthesized as early as 1853, with no recognition of its value. Aniline, or aminobenzene, was acetylated in 1852. Its medicinal use resulted from a prescription error when a Strassburg pharmacist put it in a preparation for treating a patient with a febrile reaction to intestinal parasites. It was noted to have reduced the fever. This occurred in 1886. The following year, Alfred Kast (1856-1903), of sulfonal fame, introduced phenaacetin or the ethyl ester of p-acetylamino phenol. *(Centralb Med Wiss,* Berlin, 25:145-148, 1887). This compound effectively masked the amino group by acetylation and the phenolic hydroxyl group by ethylation. The properties both of aniline and phenol were combined in the parent compound, p-amino-phenol. Thus a successful antipyretic was devised by the sharp biochemorphic skill of Kast.

Milton Silverman *(Magic in a Bottle,* New York Macmillan, 1941, pp. 185-187) tells how acetphenetidin was first prepared. Carl Duisburg (1861-1935), director of research at the Friedrich Bayer dye factory, wanted to get rid of a big pile of crude p-amino-phenol. He suggested acetylating the amino group and blocking the hydroxyl with methyl or ethyl. Large scale manufacture resulted in the safe, effective and inexpensive phenacetin. Duisberg later aided in the formation of the great I. G. Farbenindustrie and became board chairman in 1925.

It was noted that acetphenetidin reduced fever temperature by as much as 2°C within an hour or so after an oral dose of 0.2 to 0.5 gm without side effects. Animal studies showed little toxicity. Von Mering found that the drug is metabolized in part to N-acetyl-p-aminophenol, and part excreted in the urine combined with glucuronic acid *(Ther Mon, 7:577-587, 1893)*. Paul K. Smith (1908-1965) prepared a critical bibliography of acetphenetidin with 529 references, one-third of which are before 1900 *(Interscience,* New York City, 1958, 180 pp.)

Somewhile previously, however, Wilhelm Filehne (1844-1927) had introduced the more complex synthetic antipyrine as an effective antipyretic *(Ztsch Klin Med, 7:641-642, 1884)*. This had been prepared by Ludwig Knorr (1859-1921), later of Wurzburg. This resulted from Knorr's isolation of the pyrazole ring antipyrine being dimethyl phenyl pyrazoline. It was a brilliant synthesis designed to produce a useful antipyretic, and it did so. Knorr gave patent rights to the Hoeschst Company, near Frankfurt, for large scale production of antipyrine and its exploitation. It was a big factor in German drug monopoly.

Filehne then went further to make and develop the dimethyl amino derivative of antipyrine which he introduced under the tradename of Pyramidon® *(Berl Klin Wochenschr, 33:1061-1063, 1896)*. Both antipyrine and amidopyrine were early noted to be anti-inflammatory, as well as antipyretic. As such they have long since been used as analgesics in arthritis and rheumatism or congestive pain. They tend to cause agranulocytosis, so that their use is declining. A 4-butyl, 2-phenyl derivative of antipyrine has more recently been introduced by the great Swiss drug firm, J. R. Geigy A. G., under the public name, phenylbutazone. This drug has twenty-two tradenames. Chemically, it is 1,2-diphenyl-3, 5-dioxo-4-n-butyl-pyrazolidine. This drug is now widely used to relieve gout, arthritis, and rheumatic pain. It is interesting that Knorr's isolation of the pyrazole ring, in the search for a substitute for quinine, should continue to be so fruitful.

The bark and leaves of Salix, the willow, were anciently used, especially in the Eastern Mediterranean, to relieve the pain of arthritis and rheumatism. The willow leaves or bark were crushed in olive oil and applied from specially formed clay pots to painful joints. Similarly, North Amerinds used an oil pressed from wintergreen to apply to arthritic or rheumatic areas on the skin. From willow is obtained salicylic acid, and oil of wintergreen is methyl salicylate. In their historical introduction to a review of the salicylates (New Haven, Hillhouse, 1948, 380 pp, with 4093 references!), Martin Gross and Leon Greenberg discount this anti-inflammatory use of willow and wintergreen, noting internal use as a diuretic, although acknowledging use of willow leaves for gout.

My long-time friend, Maurice Tainter, has succinctly sketched the story of the development of the salicylates *(Aspirin in Modern Therapy: A Review,* New York, Sterling Drug Co., 1969, 128 pp). I can do no better than to paraphrase parts of it. Milton Silverman, in his skillful, dramatic way, recounts the same events.

In a short note, the Reverend Edward Stone first called attention in modern times to the antipyretic properties of willow preparations, especially in "anguish and intermitting fevers"—meaning malaria *(Philos Trans R Soc Lon, 53:*195, 1763). Leroux found a glucoside, salicin, in willow bark *(J Chim Med, 6:*341, 1830). After the preparation of salicylic acid from salicin by Piria in 1838, and from oil of gaultheria (wintergreen) by August André Cahours (1813-1891) in 1845, acetyl salicylic acid was made by Charles Frédéric Gerhardt (1816-1856), Professor of Chemistry at Strassburg *(Leibig's Ann, 87:*149, 1853). These advances excited no interest.

In 1874, however, Adolph Wilhelm Hermann Kolbe (1818-1884), a pupil of Wöhler, discovered a reaction, now known by his name, which enabled him easily to make large amounts of salicylic acid. Its antiseptic properties were used in the preservation of meat and milk. Its sodium salt was recognized as having antipyretic action. It seems to have been the histologist, Solomon Stricker (1834-1898) who noted its beneficial effect in acute rheumatic disorders *(Berl Klin Wochenschr, 13:*1-2, 99-103, 1876) and noted that sodium salicylate appears to be able to arrest acute rheumatic fever.

The Bayer group at Elberfeld was anxious to get a safe nonirritating derivative of salicylic acid. Heinrich Dreser (1860-1924) of Darmstadt was director of research. He was a pupil of Schmiedeberg, had been Professor of Pharmacology at Gottingen, and was a prodigious writer. One of his chemists brought him a sample of acetyl salicylic acid hoping it would be less irritating to the stomach of his father than sodium salicylate necessary to control arthritic pain. Dreser demonstrated relative lack of local irritation from acetyl salicylic acid by using gills of live goldfish. Milton Silverman tells the story dramatically. Clinical trials were successful *(Arch Ges Physiol, 76:*306-318, 1899), and with a flood of confirmatory reports, the new drug was widely exploited.

A short name was sought for acetyl salicylic acid. Dreser recalled how salicylic acid was early obtained from *Spiraea* plants and called spiric acid. The new drug was named acetyl-spiric-acid, a-spiric acid, and finally *aspirin*. It soon became the most generally used drug all over the world, after alcohol in alcoholic beverages. Only later was it realized that it does have side effects, including allergic reactions, and locally irritating action on the stomach mucosa. My good and modest friend, John C. Krantz, Jr. of Baltimore, devised a tablet of aspirin containing aluminum glycinate as a mild buffer, trademarked and exploited as Bufferin®.

The marked headache and arthritic pain-relieving properties of aspirin have resulted in its being made into many combinations, often with caffeine, sometimes with acetphenetidin. All these are distastefully advertised in all media, especially television; for over-the-counter direct sale in drug stores, or even grocery stores and supermarkets.

Aspirin remains, after alcohol, the most widely used drug, tons of it being made and sold annually. There is an interesting point about it relating to its extensive advertising as Bayer® aspirin. In a famed legal action for infringement of tradename rights, the United States Supreme Court ruled it had been over-advertised to the extent that it had become a common name. Until then, if a physician prescribed aspirin, with no designation, the pharmacist furnished Bayer Aspirin; if some other drug company's name was used, the pharmacist had to supply it, but if acetylsalicylic acid was prescribed, the pharmacist could supply any brand he may choose.

The mechanism of action of aspirin remains in dispute. It is a very effective antipyretic analgesic agent. How does it reduce fever and give relief in so many painful conditions, from head and toothache, to joint and muscle pain? It is to be noted that it is much more effective in relieving congestive pain than in alleviating traumatic pain. Morphine raises the threshold to painful stimuli; aspirin does not.

Pharmacology in the Second Half of Nineteenth Century 163

Current pharmacologic texts seem to be at a loss adequately to explain the action of the antipyretic analgesics. Most assume a central action; the analgesia the result of an interference with transmission of pain impulses between the hypothalamus and the sensory cortex. The antipyresis follow an interference with heat-regulating centers in the hypothalamus with resulting peripheral vasodilation aiding in heat dissipation, and the anti-inflammatory effect is due to hyaluronidase inhibition and to stimulation of the adrenal cortex with cortisone release. The evidence for any one of these presumed mechanisms is weak.

On the other hand, forgotten seem to be the clearcut results of experimental studies by Henry Gray Barbour (1866-1943), Professor of Pharmacology at Louisville and later at Yale. When he conducted some of his experiments at the University of Wisconsin, I helped him. His idea was simple. Provocative antigens, whether from microorganisms or otherwise, liberating histamine from cells in a rigid case, such as the skull, a tooth, a joint, or muscle in a sheath, would cause an inflammatory reaction with swelling, chiefly through fixation of water in cells. The increased pressure, distorting the blood vessels in the rigid case, would cause the sensory stimulus interpreted as pain. The antipyretic analgesics, reversing this water fixation, would relieve the pressure and thus the pain. Since these drugs are metabolized within four hours or so and excreted in the urine in combination with glucuronic acid, or glycine, the dosage would have to be repeated every four hours to maintain relief in the face of the continued presence of the provocative antigen.

This idea was extended to fevers. Here the provocative antigen might disturb water and electrolyte balance widely in cells throughout the body, even if only a small amount for each cell. The overall result, however, would be a loss of circulating water in the blood, so that the resulting hemoconcentration would prevent adequate water loss through the skin and from the lungs so that the cooling effect of evaporation therefrom would be lost and the temperature would go up. This situation would give the characteristic signs of fever, dry skin and mucous membranes, dry hot breath, scanty urine, and rise in body temperature. The antipyresis would result from the drug action in reversing this picture, pulling water out of the cells, and making it available in the blood for the usual loss through the skin and lungs with cooling by evaporation. The water shift in individual cells might be small indeed, but when the allergic reaction is generalized involving uncountable numbers of cells, the overall effect might be considerable.

This idea was put to test in a variety of animals, including cats, dogs, rats, and rabbits, with fever induced by injection of cocaine, peptone, or dead typhoid bacilli. Hemoconcentration or dilution was followed by stopwatching the rate of fall of a standardized blood drop through a mixture of brombenzene and xylene adjusted to a bit less than the specific gravity of blood. The method is exquisitely sensitive, and when standardized is remarkably accurate and reproducible. During the onset of fever one can correlate temperature rise with hemoconcentration. On administering an antipyrine analgesic drug, such as acetanalid, antipyrine, phenacetin, or aspirin, hemodilution is noted a short while before temperatures fall, or in the case of dogs, before the tongue moistens or panting occurs. So uniform were these findings that I instituted these experiments as class exercises for pharmacology students and thus collected much data on the matter. When studied clinically in patients, the same results were found. The studies were widely reported *(Am J Physiol, 59:445, 1922; J Physiol, 59:300, 1924; Am J Physiol, 67:366-378, 1924; 73:315, 1925; J Pharmacol Exp Ther, 60:224, 1937, and others)*.

It would seem that there is a significant peripheral effect of the antipyretic analgesics. The mechanism, however, still remains obscure. Anterior pituitary stimulation, with release of adrenocorticotrophic hormone, or direct action on the adrenal cortex to release cortisone, is not ruled out by Barbour's work. Nor do his findings preclude some obscure central action on hypothalaminic heat centers. Yet, they deserve consideration. Certainly with the sophisticated techniques now available, one would think that intensive study would be justified of the mechanism of action of such a widely used drug as aspirin.

A further commentary is indicated on Heinrich Dreser. He must have been impressed with the role of the acetyl group in reducing toxicity of organic compounds. With his chemists at the Bayer Company he prepared diacetylmorphine, muzzling both the alcoholic and phenolic hydroxyl groups of morphine with the acetyl grouping. This new compound was dubbed heroin, and was introduced as a safer and quicker pain reliever than morphine. It is quickly metabolized and its action is relatively brief.

When heroin was first used, it was enthusiastically acclaimed. It suppressed cough well. Within a few years, however, a veritable flood of reports appeared detailing the unpleasantness of addiction to it. On injection it made one feel fine. As the short action faded on continuing use, unpleasant feelings appeared—abdominal pains and cramps and general malaise. These were found to be quickly relieved by another dose of the drug. The cycle of viciousness was on the way; within a few years heroin was banned in all alert countries. Then it became profitable to furnish it to those who wanted a thrill, or to escape from the misery of slum living, and the drug problem was upon us.

Aspirin was not the only important salicylate devised in the latter part of the nineteenth century. Marcel von Nencki (1847-1901) made phenylsalicylate or salol in 1886, and introduced it as a mild intestinal antiseptic (which it is not). This compound is not split in the stomach, but in the alkalinity of the small intestine, it slowly is hydrolyzed to phenol and salicylic acid, which, excreted in the urine in combination with glucuronic acid and glycine, are mildly antiseptic to the urinary tract. Hermann Sahli (1856-1933) a Professor of Medicine at Berne, had much to do with the clinical introduction of salol.

The importance of salol, however, is due to its pioneering use for selective localization of drug action. As a coating for capsules, pills or tablets, it allows the drugs contained therein to pass through the stomach, and to be released in the small bowel for action or absorption there. This principle has been widely extended with pharmaceutical preparations for sustained release of drugs in the bowel in order to prolong the activity and reduce toxic reaction to a large amount of a drug.

The development of the analgesic antipyretics was one of the most important pharmacological achievements of the latter half of the nineteenth century. It all came as a result of an effort to get inexpensive, effective and safe substitutes for quinine. Karl Binz (1832-1913) of Bonn wrote much on the antipyretic action and uses of quinine and the salicylates. He realized that the salicylates lacked something inherent in quinine, namely the ability to cure malaria. The search for fully satisfactory substitutes for quinine continued.

Homeopathic Drugs

One of the major medical fallacies of the nineteenth century was the theoretical exposition of homeopathy. This was the reaction of Christian Friedrich Samuel Hahnemann (1755-1843) against the abusive polypharmacy of bleeding, sweating, purging and vomiting characteristic of the early nineteen century therapeutics. The practical effects of homeopathy in reducing violent drug therapy gradually became apparent as the nineteenth century moved along. The introduction of pure chemical compounds, with clinical use based on the results of controllable animal experimentation, was certainly the chief factor in the rise of a rational drug usage. From this position, the use of homeopathic crude drugs, in homeopathic, or infinitely small doses, was clear retrogression. At best it confirmed again the ancient Hippocratic dictum that sick people often get well regardless of drugs or other therapy. The *vis medicatrix naturae* continues to act.

Homeopathic drug use reached its high point in the latter half of the nineteenth century and then steadily dwindled away. By the end of the century, Hahnemann's theory, embodied in his *Organon der Rationellen Heilkunde* (Dresden, Arnold, 1810, 430 pp.) was an historical curiosity.

Homeopathic drugs are legion. This is due to their subjective method of proving, in the original sense of testing. The saying, "It's the exception that proves the rules," really means that it is the exception which tests the rule. All kinds of plant materials, many favored by the "Naturopaths" of the mid-America nineteenth century were chewed and ingested by homeopathic searchers who made detailed observations on the symptoms they were thought to make the researcher feel. If these symptoms were in any way similar to the symptoms reported as characteristic of a disease, the plant material, properly prepared and diluted many times (10 x meaning a hundred fold) with milk sugar was recommended for the treatment of that disease. This was based on Hahnemann's dictum *similia simili-*

bus curantur, a revival in a way of the ancient doctrine of signatures. He insisted that the dynamic effect of such drugs was greatly increased by almost infinite dilution.

Homeopathic drugs certainly did no harm. Homeopathy flourished in many European countries as well as in the U.S. The homeopathic physicians were gentle and sympathetic, in marked contrast to the often arrogant disdain of their more conventional colleagues. Practical psychotherapy played as much of a role in the success of homeopaths as the diluted crude plant drugs they used. But homeopathy gradually went into limbo as the clear-cut value of rationally developed drugs, with confirmable objective pharmacological evidence behind them, became well recognized by the end of the nineteenth century.

Modern Pharmacology

Pharmacology, as the scientific discipline concerned basically with chemically interactions in living material, began and rapidly expanded in the nineteenth century. It started with the rise of chemistry as a quantitative science. This permitted study of the direct physiological effects of pure chemical agents on living things. Promptly it led to the isolation in chemically pure, usually crystalline, form of the significantly biologically-active agents buried for centuries in empirically used crude drugs of plant, animal and mineral materials. The fundamental scientific problems delineating pharmacology as a science were outlined and explored: (1) the dose-effect relationship; (2) the question of the rates of drug absorption into, distribution through, and removal from living material; (3) the localization of the site of action of drugs; (4) the mechanisms of the action of drugs on living material, and (5) the relationship between the physiochemical constitution of a chemical compound and its biological activity.

Great practical success resulted from pharmacological effort in the nineteenth century; anesthesia and antisepsis markedly influenced surgical advance, and the economic situation regarding quinine resulted in the great benefits of the antipyretic analgesics. Some practical pharmacological successes were fortuitous, as in the introduction of the nitrites for angina pectoris. Others were remarkably deliberate, as in the development of sleep-producing drugs. These practical successes greatly improved the quality of health care, from nursing through pharmacy, dentistry, medicine and surgery, to veterinary medicine. With the rise of microbiology and the recognition of the bacterial and parasitic origin of infectious disease, correlated with the discovery of antiseptic drugs, a glimpse was given of the possibility of preventive medicine, to become public health in later years. The recognition of the dangers of drug addiction focused attention on the possible need for public regulation of drug use.

Glimpses of future development in pharmacology also came as the nineteenth century drew to a close. Radiation physics was underway and radioactive chemical were beginning to be studied. The huge field of endocrinology was beginning to open up as biologically active chemical compounds were found in various glands of vertebrate bodies. Even the necessary accessory food factors we call vitamins were beginning to be glimpsed. The vast potentialities of pharmacological study of the autonomic nervous system was beginning to be appreciated. Already in bud were what were to become the amazing fruits of chemotherapeutic effort. Biochemical advance was already suggesting the successes to be found in pharmacological study of enzymes and metabolic disorders. Not too far off was an impressive approach to Jame Blake's idea that full knowledge of the physicochemical structure of a drug would reveal information about the structure of the molecules of living material with which that drug might react.

As a result of quantitative studies in pharmacology, it was possible by the end of the 19th Century to suggest the factors which are responsible for the intensity of action of a drug on living material. It was beginning to be appreciated that the reaction between drugs and living material goes two ways: drugs alter the activity of living materials, but living material also alters drugs.

Drug effects are produced by the interaction of molecules of the drug with molecules of living material. This reaction goes along the organizational levels of living material from molecules to subcellular structures, to cells, to organs and tissues, to individuals, to societies and to environments. Yet, it became apparent that we are not able to predict from what occurs at one level what may happen at the next, except in a general way. No matter how much we learn about organs and tissues, for example, we can not tell in advance what any individual may be like, except very generally.

The factors which determine the intensity of action of a drug are: (1) the dosage expressed in molar concentrations of drug per mass of living material; (2) the ratio of the rate of absorption of the drug into the living material, and its distribution through the living material to the rate of the removal of the drug from the living material; (3) the physicochemical properties of the drug, and (4) the peculiar individual properties of the living material, such as age, metabolic or allergic state, diseased condition, sex, nutritional balance, and such. The first three factors are measurable, while the last is indeterminate and dependent upon objective judgment. The product of the first two gives the concentration of the drug in the living material at any given moment.

With all the premonition of what pharmacology as a science might become, as indicated in the nineteenth century, many amazing surprises to come were not anticipated. These came as a result of war, population pressures, cognate scientific advance, and ancient hopes. Pharmacology in the twentieth century was truly to become complex, often baffling, but increasingly interesting and challenging as its applications were to become increasingly far-reaching.

CHAPTER 11

PROGRESS AND PROMISE: TRANSITION OF PHARMACOLOGY FROM THE 19TH CENTURY INTO THE 20TH

PHARMACOLOGICAL PROGRESS TOWARD the end of the nineteenth century gave promise of such significant knowledge to come about drugs and how they work. The major pharmacological concepts in the latter part of the nineteenth century which foreshadowed much to come in the twentieth were:

1. chemotherapy from organometallic compounds through sulfa drugs to antibiotics;
2. analysis of the actions of and development of clinically useful autonomic drugs;
3. Derivation of central nervous system stimulants, depressants, and hallucinogens, with analysis of their actions, and including psychotropic drugs and the management of their abuses;
4. analysis of the actions of and development of clinically useful endocrine drugs;
5. development of clinically useful radio-opaque and radio-active diagnostic agents;
6. analysis of the actions of and development of vitamins;
7. recognition of the importance of enzyme mediation in drug action;
8. beginning of an appreciation of the social and ecological effects of chemical compounds, and
9. beginning of bureaucratic governmental control of drug use.

Chemotherapy arose as a consequence of the demonstration

of microorganisms as causes of infectious disease as made by Louis Pasteur (1822-1895) and Robert Koch (1843-1910), and as applied in surgery by Joseph Lister (1827-1912). In developing a vaccine for diphtheria, Emil Von Behring (1854-1917) introduced the technique of standardizing it against an arbitrary reference standard by biological testing. This assured reasonable uniformity in the vaccine. In this he was aided by a brilliant but sloppy chemist, Paul Ehrlich (1854-1915), who was trying to stain microorganisms and the cells of various tissues. In this effort he was successful.

With Koch, Ehrlich thought of finding a stain which might be poisonous to bacteria without harming living cells. The common fear of arsenic trioxide as a poison suggested combining arsenic into an organic molecule which might selectively stain bacteria. The simplest was p-aminophenylarsonate, the sodium salt of which was named Atoxyl, since it was relatively non-toxic in comparison with arsenic trioxide. Atoxyl was found to be highly poisonous to trypanosomes, the causative agent of African sleeping sickness. Koch used Atoxyl to treat this disease, but it was not fully satisfactory.

In an effort to improve upon Atoxyl, Ehrlich set out to make as many related arsenical compounds as possible. Fortunately, he now had his own laboratory. The story is vividly told by Milton Silverman in his exciting *Magic in a Bottle* (New York, Macmillan, 1941, 332 pp.).

Ehrlich found several arsenical compounds which would kill trypanosomes in rats without injuring the host animals. His methods for estimating the therapeutic indices of these drugs were statistically crude, being based on doses which would give three out of five cures or three out of five deaths. One compound, the 606th of his series, 3,3'-diamino-4,4'-dihydroxyarsenobenzene dihydrochloride, was audaciously tried on human syphilis on the tenuous basis of a similarity between spirochetes, the causative germs of syphilis, and trypanosomes. Ehrlich was lucky: it worked. Salvarsan, as the compound was called, was the first wonder drug of the twentieth century.

Emil von Behring's studies on diphtheria and tetanus antitoxins were published with Shibasaburo Kitasato (1852-1931) in brief notes in 1890 (*Deutsch Med Wochenshr, 16*:1113-1114, 1145-1148). Ehrlich's work on standardization of vaccines came in 1897 (*Klin Jahresb, 6*:297-326). In this he first proposed his side chain theory to explain the bactericidal action of vaccines and chemicals. A summary of Ehrlich's studies on the chemotherapy of syphilis was published with Sahachiro Hata (1873-1938) in 1910 (*Die Experimentellen Chemotherapie der Spirillosen*, Berlin, Springer).

Ehrlich's development of staining methods for living tissue began as early as 1886 (*Deutsch Med Wochenshr, 12*:49-52), but his development of aniline stains for cells and bacteria came a decade earlier (*Arch Mikr Anat, 13*:263-277, 1877). Koch's clinical studies on the management of trypanosomiasis appeared in 1898 (*Reise-Bericht über Rinderpest, Tsetse-oder Surra krankheit*, Berlin, Springer). From these nineteenth century efforts at treating infectious diseases evolved the vast chemotherapeutic successes of the twentieth century.

The pharmacology of the autonomic nervous system developed along with expanding knowledge of its embryology, anatomy and physiology. Claude Bernard (1813-1878) demonstrated the physiological significance of the sympathetic nervous system with his discovery of the vasomotor responses to stimulation of sympathetic nerve trunks (*Compt Rend Acad Sci, 47*:245-253, 1858), while Walter Gaskell (1847-1914) showed the nature of the action of the vagus nerves in slowing the heart (*Philos Trans R Soc, 173:* 993-1033, 1882).

John Newport Langley (1852-1925) clearly differentiated the sympathetic and parasympathetic aspects of the autonomic nervous system, showing their complementary and often antagonistic physiological and pharmacological reactions. Whereas activation of the sympathetic system is followed by increased blood pressure and heart rate, with bronchial and digestive tract relaxation, activation of the parasympathetic system is followed by decreased blood pressure and heart rate with increased tone of bronchial and intestinal muscles. He found that nicotine paralyzes ganglionic synapses when applied to them as they occur in the autonomic nervous system. He thus was able to locate the characteristic short postganglionic fibers in the parasympathetic system as well as the long postganglionic fibers typical of the sympathetic system. Langley's great work, begun in the last years of the nineteenth century, culminated in the twentieth in his classic, *The Autonomic Nervous System,* (Cambridge University Press, 1921).

Among drugs, pilocarpine and physostigmine, alkaloids from natural sources long used in African folklore, were recognized as activating the parasympathetic system, while the action of the long-used European belladonna, and its active ingredient, atropine, were explained on the basis of inhibition of parasympathetic nerves. The biomedical actions of pilocarpine and physostigmine can be antagonized by atropine, and vice versa. These three drugs are toxic if taken in excess.

Meanwhile, George Oliver (1841-1915) and Edward Sharpey-Schäffer (1850-1935) had demonstrated the presence of a blood-pressure-raising substance in the medulla of adrenal glands *(J Physiol, 18:*230-276, 1895). This substance was isolated by John Jacob Abel (1857-1938) and Albert C. Crawford (1869-1921), with attempts to characterize it chemically *(Bull Johns Hopkins Hosp, 8:*151-157, 1897). They called it epinephrine. But Jokichi Takamine (1854-1922) determined its chemical constitution and patented it under the name adrenaline *(Am J Pharm, 73:*523-531, 1901). It was recognized as an amine.

Meticulous studies on the chemical structure and biological action of amines were undertaken by George Barger (1878-1939) and Henry Dale (1875-1968) to culminate in a classical pharmacological report issued in 1910 *(J Physiol, 41:*19-59). This was the basis for extensive pharmacological studies made through the twentieth century on amphetamines and catecholamines. Epinephrine and its demethylated derivative, norepinephrine, were gradually realized to be a chemical mediators of sympathetic action. Chemical mediation in the parasympathetic system was slower to be appreciated. The work of Reid Hunt (1870-1948) on choline derivatives pointed the way *(J Pharmacol Exp Ther, 1:* 303-309, 1909).

The discovery of epinephrine aroused interest in the possibility of the release of other kinds of chemicals from other ductless glands. The thyroid gland had long attracted clinical interest through its association with goiter. Ashes of seaweed had been a folk-remedy for goiter. These ashes were found to contain iodine. This chemical itself was first used against goiter by Jean François Coindet (1774-1834), as reported in 1820 (*Ann Chim Phys, 15:* 49-59).

Surgical removal of thyroid glands was noted to be followed by thickened skin and physical sluggishness. George R. Murray (1865-1939) reported success in 1891 in treating myxedema, as the condition was called, by injections of an extract of thyroid gland (*Br Med J, 2:*796-797). Studies on thyroid extract by Eugen Baumann, 1846-1896) showed it to contain iodine. (*Ztsch Physiol Chem, 21:*319-330, 1895). He isolated an iodine-containing amino acid from thyroid, much later to be characterized chemically as thyroxine.

In endocrine pharmacology, even the brilliant contributions of James B. Collip (1892-1965) on the isolation of parathormone, the active principle of the parathyroid glands which regulates blood calcium levels (*J Biol Chem, 63:*395-438, 1925), was anticipated in part by Eugene Gley (1857-1930) more than three decades earlier (*Compt Rend Soc Biol, 43:*841-847, 1891).

Although Claude Bernard (1813-1875) discovered the glycogenic function of the liver (*Arch Gen Med, 18:*303-319, 1848), and the digestive function of pancreatic juice (*Compt Rend Soc Biol, 1:*99-115, 1850), and had invented the term *internal secretion* in reference to the glycogenic activity of the liver (*Compt Rend Acad Sci, 41:*461-469, 1855), he nevertheless missed the function of the pancreas in regulating blood sugar. This was demonstrated by Joseph Mering (1849-1908) and Oscar Minkowski (1858-1931) by showing that diabetes mellitus follows removal of the pancreas (*Arch Exp Path Pharmakol, 26:*371-387, 1890). Yet it was another three decades before Frederich G. Banting (1891-1941) and Charles H. Best (1899-....) succeeded in isolating the active principle, insulin from the pancreas and in starting the successful treatment of diabetes mellitus with it (*J Lab Clin Med, 7:*251-266, 1922).

Again, several decades went by before there was satisfactory exploitation of the discovery that removal of the pituitary body is followed by a disturbance in water and mineral metabolism. This was shown by Giulio Vassali (1862-1912) in 1892 (*Riv Sper Freniat, 18:*525-561). Extracts of the posterior pituitary were studied by Henry Dale who noted their uterine effects *(Biochem J, 4:*427-447, 1909). It was another decade or so before anterior and posterior pituitary extracts were adequately studied, or characterized chemically. They are complex proteins or polypeptides.

Sex hormones were also beginning to be studied toward the end of the nineteenth century. Charles Edward Brown-Sequard (1817-1894), who worked for a while in the U.S., created quite a sensation by injecting testicular extracts for rejuvenation *(Arch Physiol, 1:*651-658, 1889). It came to little at the time, but the general idea led to the isolation of the ovarian hormone, estrogen, by Edgar Allen (1892-1943) and Edward Doisy (1893-....) in 1923 *(JAMA, 81:*819-821, 1923). Chemical characterization came a decade later, with recognition of the steroid conformation of the molecules of the sex hormones and their relation to other sterols, including those which inhibit ovulation, ("the Pill").

Even the blood-pressure-raising factor, renin from kidneys, which is currently so important as shown by Irvine Page (1901-....), was anticipated in the closing years of the nineteenth century. The great Finnish physiologist, Robert Adolf Tigerstedt (1853-1923) first demonstrated in 1898 that renin is produced by kidneys and secreted into the blood circulation by way of the renal veins *(Skand Arch Physiol, 8:*223-271).

Drugs acting on the brain and central nervous system were being well developed in the latter part of the nineteenth century. Oscar Liebreich (1839-1908) had introduced chloral hydrate as a sleep-producing drug in 1869 *(Arch Deutsch Ges Psychiat, 16:* 237), while Vincenzo Cervello (1854-1919) had introduced paraldehyde for the same purpose in 1884 *(Arch Ital Biol, 6:*113-134). Wilhelm Filehne (1844-1929) developed antipyrine in 1884 as a substitute for quinine in reducing fever *(Ztsch Klin Med, 7:*641-642), and in 1896 introduced amidopyrine for the same purpose *(Berl Klin Wochenchr, 33:*1061-1063). Both were recognized as central nervous system depressants, as was sulfonal, developed by Eugen Baumann and Alfred Kast (1856-1903) in 1888 (*Berl Klin Wochenschr, 25*:309-314).

The central depressant effects of urea derivatives were recognized by the great biochemist, Emil Fischer (1852-1919) in 1896 (*Ber Deutsch Chem Ges, 28*:2473-2480), and this was exploited into the development of barbituric acid derivatives, with Joseph Mering in 1903 (*Ther Gegenw, 44*:97-101). The initial one was Veronal, later given the public name, barbital, to be followed by its phenyl derivative, Luminal. The patenting of these compounds, as in the case of Salvarsan®, had much to do with the phenomenal rise of the German drug industry during the first part of the twentieth century, and its association with dye and explosive manufacturing. A head start on World War I! The exploitation of barbital derivatives continues to this day.

While the central nervous stimulating effects of caffeine and its chemical relatives was recognized in the late nineteenth century, as was also the case of strychnine and epinephrine, little was done about developing new drugs until Gordon Alles (1901-1963) in our San Francisco laboratory undertook to make a synthetic substitute for epinephrine used in the treatment of asthma. This effort took him back to the gold mine of Barger and Dale's 1910 classic, and from his skill came amphetamine. This was soon realized to be a potent central nervous system stimulant. It never occurred to us that it might be badly abused. I've told this story in detail in *The Amphetamines* (Springfield, Thomas, 1958, 167 pp).

Among the chemical relatives of epinephrine and ephedrine is mescaline. This had been isolated from peyote or mescal by Arthur Heffter (1860-1925) and was studied by him and by the great toxicologist, Louis Lewin (1850-1929). They noted its hallucinogenic properties (*Arch Exp Pathol Pharmakol, 40*:418-425, 1897). Henry Havelock Ellis (1859-1939), the great pioneer of sexual psychology, also noted the hallucinogenic properties of mescaline (*Lancet 1*:1540-1542, 1897), as did S. Weir Mitchell (1829-1914), the great Philadelphia neurologist (*Br Med J, 2*: 1625-1629, 1896). Only decades later were these observations to be exploited by the rebellious youth of the 1960's.

The central nervous system disturbances of ergot had been recognized in medieval Europe in connection with the mass poisonings resulting from eating bread from smutty rye. The smut was the amazing fungus, ergot, from which the alkaloid, ergotoxine was isolated by Barger and Dale in 1906 (*Br Med J, 2:* 1792). But it was the great Swiss chemist, Arthur Stoll (1887-1971), who showed that ergot alkaloids, antagonists to epinephrine, are derivatives of lysergic acid (*Schw Arch Neurol Psychiat, 60:*279-324, 1947). This led to the synthesis of its diethylamide derivative, LSD and the accidental discovery of its powerful hallucinogenic action by Albert Hoffman (1906-....) and the resulting recognition of its abuse (*Sandoz J Med, 3:*117-124, 1955).

The hallucinogenic effects of certain tropical mushrooms and of the seeds of bind-weed, *Rivea corumbosa* (Ololiuque), have been known in folklore for ages. Yet the active principles therein were not investigated until Hoffman clarified them by showing a tryptamine derivative, psilocybin, to be the active agent in the Psylocybe mushrooms and a lysergic acid amide to be the active agent in the latter.

Similarly, snake-root, mentioned by the ancient Hindus and by Dioscorides in our first century as an agent for the relief of mania, was not systematically investigated until well into the twentieth century. The plant was named *Rauwolfia* in honor of Leonard Rauwolf, a sixteenth century botanizing physician. From it was obtained the alkaloid, reserpine, which is amazingly effective in quieting manic disturbance. This alkaloid contains, as a part of its molecule, tryptamine, which is closely related to 5-hydroxytryptamine (serotonin) occurring in nervous tissue and acts in part by releasing from nerves the catechol amines, norepinephrine and epinephrine.

After many centuries we can begin to explain how many anciently used plant remedies act. This is largely due to the chemical methodologies developed in the nineteenth century for the extraction, isolation, purification and identification of the biologically active substances hidden away in the gums, resins, tannins, celluloses and chlorophylls of the natural products.

One of the most significant of biomedical advances in the

twentieth century was the recognition of the effects of radiant energy on living things. This included many applications of radiant energy to diagnosis and treatment of disease. The effects of sunlight were well appreciated in antiquity, even to the recognition that too much exposure might be harmful. The arrows of Apollo both healed and harmed.

In the nineteenth century came recognition of the catalytic action of sunlight on growth of plants and the discovery of the wide range of radiant energy from short wave X-rays, through ultraviolet, visible spectrum, and infrared, to the long radio waves. Wavelengths of radiant energy and vibration frequencies came to be measured. Antoine Henri Becquerel (1852-1908) discovered radioactivity, and Pierre (1859-1906) and Marie Curie (1867-1934) isolated radium (*Compt Rend Acad Sci, 127*:175-178, 1898). And Wilhelm Conrad Roentgen (1845-1923) accidentally found X-rays and opened a whole new field of technology (*Ueber Eine Neue Art Von Strahlen, S.B. Phys. Med. Ges. Wurzburg,* 1895, 132-141).

Roentgen-ray visualization of the alimentary tract, using radio-opaque bismuth and later barium salts, was undertaken by Walter Bradford Cannon (1871-1945) in 1898 (*Am J Physiol, 1:* 359-382), while still a medical student at Harvard. This was the beginning of extensive development in the twentieth century of radio-opaque drugs of many kinds for X-ray visualization of body cavities and even blood vessels. The extent of the development has been well documented by my long-time colleague, Peter K. Knoefel (*Radiocontrast Agents,* Oxford, Pergamon Press, 1971, 2 vols. 785 pp.).

Cannon's work was of the utmost importance. It led eventually to the recognition of many chemical and nervous factors involved in maintaining an internal steady state in living bodies. This had been noted by Claude Bernard (*Leçons sur les Phénomènes de la Vie,* Paris Baillière, 1878, 2 vols.). It was carefully detailed by Cannon in his concept of homeostasis as described in his book, *The Wisdom of the Body* (New York Norton, 1932). The feedback control mechanisms Cannon outlined were developed by his mathematician-colleague, Norbert Wiener (1904-

1964), into what was called cybernetics, which became the basis of computers. (*Cybernetics, or Control and Communication in Animals and Machines,* New York, Wiley, 1948, 193 pp.).

Cannon was well prepared for his endeavor. He grew up in Prairie du Chien, Wisconsin, where his boyhood hero had been William Beaumont (1785-1853). Beaumont was the fascinating U.S. Army surgeon who treated the fur trader, Alexis St. Martin, whose abdomen was shot open in a fracas at Mackinnaw. The wound healed, to Beaumont's surprise, leaving an opening through which one could watch the movements and secretions of the stomach. This Beaumont did, keeping copious notes, while at Fort Crawford at Prairie du Chien. Beaumont observed the influence of emotional changes on stomach motion and secretion. Beaumont's study appeared after long labor (*Experiments and Observations on the Gastric Juice, and the Physiology of Digestion,* Plattsburgh, Allen, 1833, 280 pp.).

Cannon knew Beaumont's work thoroughly. When Roentgen described X-rays, Cannon realized he had a way to study the movement of the entire alimentary tract in animals and proceeded to do so. He observed emotional changes on the activity of the gut in cats and related some of this to release of epinephrine from the adrenal medulla. Beaumont's work also stimulated the initiation of the remarkable studies of Ivan Pavlov (1849-1925) on digestion and then on conditioned reflexes.

Cannon followed intestinal motility by means of radio-opaque balls and solutions, revealed by X-rays on a fluorescent screen. He traced what he saw on toilet paper. Rolls of his tracings may be seen in the Museum in Prairie du Chien.

The beginning of radio-opaque diagnostic drugs is an amazing instance of how prepared minds can take advantage of happenstance and crash through. But Cannon paid. His hands became badly burned by the X-rays. It remains necessary to warn repeatedly of the dangers of radio-contrast drugs used for diagnosis, as well as of the harm that may come from handling radioactive compounds in metabolic studies.

Another great biomedical development of the twentieth century has been the isolation, chemical identification, pharmacological study and use of vitamins. Again, the beginnings of vitamin use go back several centuries. Balduisius Ronsseus (1525-1597) described scurvy among seamen and how they cured themselves by eating oranges and lemons *(Scorbito,* Amsterdam, Nutius, 1564).

James Lind (1716-1794) usually is credited with introducing lime and lemon juice into British navy dietaries *(A Treatise of the Scurvy,* Edinburgh, Sands, 1753). Although British seamen were derided as "limeys," they no longer suffered from scurvy. It was not until nearly two centuries later that Albert Szent-Gyorgi (1893-....) isolated ascorbic acid *(Biochem J,* 22:1387-1409, 1928) and Tadeus Reichstein (1897-....) synthesized it *Helv Chim Acta, 16*:1019-1033, 1933). Now Vitamin C, as it is commonly called, is one of the most popularly used drugs. It does help to maintain an optimum redox potential, being a relatively strong reducing compound.

Another ancient dietary deficiency disease is beri-beri, mentioned in old Chinese writings and described by Jacobus Bontius (1592-1631) in his *De Medicina Indorum* (Leyden, 1642). Kanehiro Takaki (1849-1915) associated it with a polished rice diet, and by introducing whole unpolished rice into the Japanese Navy, he got rid of beri-beri. *(Trans Sei-I-Kwai,* Tokyo, *4*:29-39, 1885).

What is it in rice polishings that prevents beri-beri? Christian Eijkman (1858-1930) tried to find out. He produced the disease experimentally by feeding a diet of polished rice alone to chickens and cleared the symptoms by adding rice polishings *(Genask T Nederl Indie, 30*:295, 1890). It was not until well into the twentieth century that clues began to be found which led eventually to the isolation of Vitamin B_1. Casimir Funk (1884-1969), who coined the word *vitamine,* thinking these accessory food factors might be amines, achieved partial isolation *(J Physiol, 43:* 395-400, 1911).

Full isolation, identification, and subsequent synthesis was achieved by Robert R. Williams (1886-1965), a Bell Telephone scientist of a missionary family *(J Am Chem Soc, 58*:1504-1505, 1936). Williams was a modest, quiet man who lived in Roselle,

New Jersey, where I grew up. I passed his home and often watched him, intent over beakers and test-tubes on a bench in his basement. I thought he was some kind of a wizard: He was. From tons of rice polishings he finally extracted a crystalline substance which he named thiamine. The big Merck drug factory in Rahway, New Jersey, aided greatly through the enlightened wisdom of George Merck (1894-1957) and his enthusiasm presently made his company a world leader in the production of vitamins.

The existence of accessory food factors in addition to the necessity for carbohydrates, fats and proteins, was first demonstrated by a student, N. Lunin, in the laboratory of Gustav Bunge (1844-1920). Lunin (about whom I cannot find anything) prepared synthetic diets of sugars, fats and proteins and showed that animals cannot live on such a chemically pure diet (*Ztscr Physiol Chem, 5*:31-39, 1881). Nothing came of this scientific demonstration of the necessity for accessory food factors, if life is to be maintained, until decades later. It was then confirmed by Frederick Gowland Hopkins (1861-1947) in 1912 (*J Physiol, 44*:425-460).

The existence of other vitamins was foreshadowed earlier than our nineteenth century. Rickets had been described by Francis Glisson (1597-1677) in the seventeenth century (*De Rachitide*, London, Du-gardi, 1650). Cod-liver oil was first reported to be useful in clearing rickets by D. Schutte (no information) in 1824 (*Arch Med Erfahr, 2*:79-92). Nearly a century later, Elmer V. McCollum (1879-1967) reported the presence in fats of an accessory factor necessary for growth (*J Biol Chem, 23*:181-246, 1913) which was called *fat-soluble A*. Vitamin D, also fat soluble, was recognized as anti-rachitic by Harry Steenbock of Wisconsin in 1921 (*J. Biol Chem, 47*:89-109). Later, Steenbock showed that ultra-violet radiation can induce calcifying properties in lipids (*J Biol Chem, 62*:209-216, 1924), thus confirming scientifically the comment of Vitruvius, the Augustan Roman architect, that sunlight is necessary to prevent rickets.

Robert Williams later showed that there are several vitamins in the water-soluble B complex (*J Biol Chem, 78*:311-322, 1928). Soon the fat-soluble vitamin saga would be filled out by my colleague, Herbert McLean Evans (1882-1971) with Vitamin E (*JAMA, 81*:889-982, 1923), and by Henrik Dam (1895-....) with Vitamin K, an anti-hemorrhagic factor (*Biochem Ztsch, 215*:475-492, 1929).

Enzymes are increasingly recognized as necessary factors in the biological activity of drugs as a result of their role in various metabolic processes, such as oxidation, reduction, dehydrogenation, demethylation, and in hydrolysis. Much of enzymatic activity was foreshadowed in studies on digestion, such as that by Theodore Schwann (1810-1882) in the discovery of pepsin for the digestion of protein in the stomach (*Arch Anat Physiol, 1836:* 90-138). This was a consequence of Beaumont's studies. Trypsin from the pancreas for digestion of protein in the intestines was discovered by Aleksander I. Danilewski (1838-1900) in 1862 *(Arch Pathol Anat, 25*:279-307).

Much interest in ferments, or enzymes, was aroused by the many reports by Louis Pasteur (1822-1895) in lactic fermentation and on the difference between fermentation in the presence and absence of oxygen (*Compt Rend Acad Sci, 56*:1189-1194, 1863). John Tyndall (1820-1893) reported on fermentation or enzyme action in relation to disease, and he noted that molds or fungi kill bacteria (*Essays*, London, Longmans, Green & Co., 1881). Tyndall had noted the bacteriostatic action of the fungus penicillium as early as 1877 (*Philos Trans R Soc, 166*:27-74). It was the rediscovery of this effect decades later by Alexander Fleming (1881-1955) that ushered in the current era of antibiotics (*Br J Exp Pathol, 10*:226-236, 1929).

Current interest in enzymes was aroused by the report in 1900 by Joseph Hoeing Kastle (1864-1919) and Arthur S. Loevenhart (1878-1929), later my mentor, on the reversibility of the action of lipase, a fat-splitting enzyme. Such reversibility in a chemical process is to be expected under mass action principles. Kastle and Loevenhart went on to study oxidases and biological oxidation, and the huge enzyme field in pharmacology went wide open.

Already by the nineteenth century drugs were being appreciated as having potential social dangers. The opium excesses of Samuel Taylor Coleridge (1772-1834) and Thomas De Quincy

(1785-1859) shocked the English. De Quincy's *Confessions of an Opium Eater* (1821) was, I think, a deliberately sensational account. It did reinforce British sentiment against the individual and social dangers of drugs. Certainly European society had its fill of misery from abuse of alcoholic beverages. The French decadents of the nineteenth century set an unwholesome example of alcohol and drug abuse, which carried into our twentieth century.

Most cultures had controlled potential abuse of hallucinogenic crude plant drugs like mushrooms and peyote by investing them with a religious aura and socializing their ritualistic use. Yet, even the strict Muslims had their troubles with the abuse of cannabis in hashish smoking.

These social experiences with drug abuse prepared the way for wide effort of social control of drug abuse in our twentieth century. This ranged from outright prohibition (with resulting corruptive racketeering) to intensive economic and educational effort. But socially we learn slowly. Each generation, it seems, has to learn the hard way.

Homicidal use of poisons, as with arsenic trioxide by the Borgias in the Renaissance, gradually came under reasonable social control as means of identification were developed for inorganic poisons and for alkaloids. The rapid rise of Toxicology in the nineteenth century prepared the way for effective control of poisonous chemicals in our twentieth century, whether in agriculture, industry, or warfare.

Effective writing on toxicology began with Nicander (185-135 BC) whose classic *Theriaca* remained popular until the seventeenth century. In the nineteenth century, Mathieu Joseph Orfila (1787-1853) prepared a widely used text on toxicology (*Traite des Poisons* Paris, 2 vols., 1818). In English, Robert Christison (1797-1882) dramatized toxicology in his *Treatise on Poisons* (A. Black, Edinburgh, 1829). James Marsh (1794-1840) took the mystery from arsenical poisoning with his sensitive and accurate test (*Edin Philos J, 21*:229-236, 1836). These were supplemented by later texts from the U.S. dealing with medical jurisprudence and toxicology. Lewis Lewin (1850-1929), the brilliant German toxicologist, could afford to become historical and ethnological in our twentieth century. His classic writings are *"Die Gifte in der Weltgeschichte"* (Berlin, Springer, 1920), and *Die Pfeilgifte* (Leipzig, Barth, 1923).

A classic start for industrial toxicology came with Bernardino Ramazzini (1633-1714), whose *De Morbis Artificum* (Capponi, Mutinae, 1700) was the first systematic consideration of occupational diseases. It was not until another century that it was surpassed, and then by a monumental work by Ludwig Hirt (1844-1907) in his *Die Krankheiten der Arbeiter* in four volumes (Hirt, Breslau, 1871-1878). In our twentieth century came Thomas Oliver (1853-1942) with his *Dangerous Trades* (London, Murray, 1902), and our own beloved Alice Hamilton (1869-1968) with her classic *Industrial Poisons in USA* (New York, Macmillan, 1925).

Snake poisoning, though feared from antiquity, was not systematically investigated until the eighteenth century, when Felice Fontana (1720-1805) issued his *Richerche Fisiche sopra il Veleno* (Lucca, Guisti, 1767). This was extended to snakes of India by Joseph Fayrer (1824-1909) in his *Thanatophidia of India* (London, Churchill, 1872), and by Silas Weir Mitchell (1829-1914) and Edward Reichert (1855-1915) to include New World species in their *Venoms of Poisonous Serpents* (Washington, Smithsonian Inst., 1886) Thomas R. Fraser (1841-1919) prepared the first anti-venom serum *(Br Med J, 1:*1309-1311, 1895).

Thus, significant nineteenth century studies on the toxicology of snake venoms led directly to the practical applications of antivenoms in our twentieth century, as illustrated in the Berkeley Symposium on *Venoms* (Amer. Asso. Adv. Sci., Washington, D.C. 1956, 467 pp., edited by Eleanor E. Buckley and Nandor Porges). Expanding knowledge of the proteins in snake venoms has been well reviewed by Jesus M. Jimenez-Porras *(Ann Rev Pharmacol, 8:*299-318, 1968).

Chemical warfare is a complicated and controversial matter. Much information on the effects of inhaling various gases was obtained during the nineteenth century, especially in anesthesia. Much of this knowledge was well summarized by Claude Bernard

(1813-1878) in his famed *Leçcons sur les Anesthesiques et sur l'Asphyxie* (Paris, Baillière, 1875). Chlorine had been used by inhalation for treating respiratory disease shortly after its isolation by Humphrey Davy (1778-1827) around 1813. This was the first poison gas used by the Germans in World War I. They developed the highly toxic *mustard gas,* dichlor-diethyl sulfide, from the inhalation anesthetic agent, diethyl oxide, or ordinary ether. My own observations on war gases were summarized in 1944, with my colleague David Marsh (*Ann Intern Med, 20*:376-389).

Lead is everywhere, and always potentially dangerous as a result of chronic ingestion. Its dangers were recognized by Vitruvius, the Augustan architect of Rome, when he cautioned against using lead pipes for conducting water, or against using lead cooking utensils. Benjamin Franklin (1706-1790) noted lead colic and palsy from drinking rum distilled through lead pipes in *An Essay on the West-India Dry-Gripes,* which he printed in 1745 for Thomas Cadwalader (1708-1779). Nothing much more was discovered regarding lead poisoning and its effective treatment until the long, careful study made by Robert A. Kehoe (1893-....) **at** the Laboratory of Applied Physiology at the University of Cincinnati, established by Charles Franklin Kettering (1876-1958) who had developed tetraethyl lead and wanted to control its potential toxicity.

Finally, it is to be noted that bureaucratic control of drug use began to develop in the nineteenth century, to reach overwhelming proportions in our time. This began with efforts at self-policing undertaken by physicians in the issuance of pharmacopeias which were given legal validity. This was to assure purity and uniformity of drugs offered to physicians by pharmacists.

The first pharmacopeia seems to have been *Pharmacorum Omnium* (Norimbergae, 1546), compiled by that brilliant youth, Valerius Cordus (1515-1544). The Royal College of Physicians issued the *Pharmacopeia Londinensis* in 1618. The first French pharmacopeia was *Codex Medicamentarius,* issued in Paris in 1638. These were revised at various intervals. The *Pharmacopeia of the United States of America* first appeared in 1820 and was revised every ten years. Gradually its function was almost completely taken over in our twentieth century by the very bureaucratic and often arbitrarily authoritarian Food and Drug Administration.

The FDA officials are simply doing their duty as they see it. They are following the law, but the law under which they operate is poor. Like most laws, it deals only in absolutes. It implies that to be approved for use, a drug must be absolutely safe and absolutely effective. There is no such drug. Gaussian distribution inevitably applies; if millions of people take the same dose of a drug, there may be some who may die of the drug as well as some on whom the drug will have no effect whatsoever.

FDA policy is costing vast sums of money in the attempt to develop worthwhile new drugs. The consumers are the ones who finally pay, and the costs of medical care continue to rise.

During the nineteenth century, thousands of new and useful drugs were introduced. The winnowing of time has eliminated many from use. Always the effort has been to improve drugs, so that they would be safer, more effective, easier to prepare and to administer, and inexpensive. Experimentation on new drugs was carefully handled by responsible pharmacologists and clinicians. Gradually, however, elaborate testing methods developed, and in the twentieth century they tended to become excessive. Now complicated protocols for drug testing include double-blind and triple-blind techniques with extensive precautions to avoid harm to anyone.

All this is necessary these days. It was only vaguely comprehended in the nineteenth century. Yet, there is evidence of continual but slow improvement in our understandings of drugs and of the biological applications of chemicals. With continual checking by experience, social benefit from the use of drugs or chemicals, whether in the health professions, in agriculture and agronomy, or in pest control, seems to increase. The process has been steadily accelerating. By the nineteenth century the major pathways to future benefits from drugs and chemicals had become clear.

Into our twentieth century pharmacology came with a rush. Its complex story will not be easy to tell. It is simply too vast, with too many keen and competent scientists involved, to be easily comprehended. Bit by bit, we add to the huge jigsaw puzzle and wonder what it is all about. Some of us will have to try to put some of the bits together. We need library as well as laboratory pharmacologists, and we need ever-increasing wisdom if we are to understand what it is all about and how we may use it to our advantage and for the welfare of our world.

It is interesting to note how often current drug or chemical problems were long ago anticipated. Several have been discussed in connection with industrial and environmental pollutants, and even with vitamins.

Pest control, even to human pests, is currently a live issue; yet its origins go back centuries. Sulfur was burned in casks or houses to fumigate them as early as Roman times. Fire-balls of sulfur and salt-petre (KNO_3) were used in warfare, as were lime and boiling oil. Fighting with chemicals was extensive in World War I. Simple procedures for reducing injury to civilians by war gases in World War II were offered by me for aid to physicians.

War gases, like many other potentially poisonous chemicals, can have a socially beneficial aspect. One of them, mustard gas (dichlorethyl sulfide) developed into a "nerve gas" (dichlorethyl amide), which was found, as a cytotoxin, to be useful in treating cancers.

On the other hand, pharmacology is now developing so rapidly amazing new types of chemicals are coming into prominence because of their potential significance for our welfare. Among them are the antihistaminics, prepared by Daniel Bovet (1907 .....) And a multitude of enzymes, and of biogenic amines. And cyclic adenosine monophosphate, with its broad biological activity as shown by Earl W. Sutherland (1915-1974). And the ubiquitous prostaglandins, whose pharmacological activities were first revealed by Ulf Svante Von Euler (1905-....) in 1934 (*Arch Exper Path Pharmakol, 175:*78-84). Note the volume number: now it is around 300, so quickly is pharmacological knowledge expanding. How may we comprehend it? Eugene Garfield, a keen documentalist, is showing some ways in the services of his Institute for Scientific Information.

APPENDED NOTES

The recent opening of the People's Republic of China to visiting physicians and scientists has permitted an assessment of the attempt to unite traditional drug practices with modern Western drug technology. The Chinese people have access in drug stores and clinics both to anciently used traditional drugs and to new scientifically developed drugs.

With public health and sanitation at a high level, there is little use for chemotherapeutic agents, such as antibiotics. There is close personal rapport between druggists and patients. Physicians tell patients fully of the conditions confronting them and of the drugs appropriate to be used. Placebos are never given. There is thus little chance for the sort of clinical pharmacology, with its elaborate statistical control, which is popular in USA. Double blind clinical trials of drugs would not be tolerated in China.

Being a practical people, the Chinese are well content with the safety and efficacy of the hundreds of crude drugs of plant, animal and mineral origin available to them from the time-tested pages of the Pen T'sao.

Bernard Read (1887-1949), formerly Professor of Pharmacology at Peking Union Medical College, and Director of the Lester Institute of Medical Research in Shanghai, has translated 26 chapters of Pen T'sao devoted to plant drugs, as compiled by Li Shih-Chen (1518-1593). There are 876 entries of plant drugs in the book (*Chinese Plant and Vegetable Drugs*, Hong Kong University Press, 1966, 750 pp.), with cross indices to scientific and Chinese names, and to general and clinical data on the drugs.

In 1974, a group of USA pharmacologists, headed by Louis Lasagna, the keen pharmacologist at the University of Rochester, New York, spent several weeks studying Chinese herbal pharmacology in China. Their report is comprehensive, and should be published. They were favorably impressed. They felt that centuries of cumulated experience by the Chinese on the safety and effectiveness of the crude drugs they used is adequate to justify their use.

In spite of the exaggerated interest in acupuncture in USA, this group found it to be little used in China. They noted that

Chinese therapy is directed toward the prompt return of the sick to normal health. Drug use in surgery is chiefly with anesthetics, with much respect for the traditional teachings of Hua-Tu, a legendary surgeon of centuries ago. He is reputed to have used hemp (cannabis) in wine as an anesthetic agent.

An interesting well-illustrated *History of Chinese Medical Science* has been issued by C. Y. Chen (Chinese Medical Institute, Hong Kong, 1969, 133 pp.). From this it is clear that the practical aspects of the use of drugs far outweigh such theoretical concepts as may be associated with them. The Chinese seem ever to be a practical people, oriented toward concrete experience rather than toward theoretical abstractions. Their language reflects this empiricism.

* * * * *

Many scholarly and well documented historical studies relating to pharmacology have appeared in the past few years, and fully deserve noting, at least for additional reading.

In *Bulletin of the History of Medicine:* W. F. Bynum on "Chemical Structure and Pharmacological Action" (44: 497-517, 1970); T. F. Brunner on "Marijuana Use in Ancient Greece and Rome" (47: 344-355, 1973); E. Lomax on "Uses and Abuses of Opiates in 19th Century England" (47: 167-176, 1973); T. Rothman on "De Laguna's Commentaries on Hallucinogenic Drugs" (46: 562-567, 1972), and J. Stannard on "Greco-Roman Materia Medica in Medieval Germany" (46: 455-468, 1972).

In *Journal of the History of Medicine:* Martin Levey on "The Pharmacological Table of ibn Biklarish" (26: 413-421, 1971); Sami Hamarneh on "Tenth-Century Arabic Medical Therapy" (27: 65-79, 1972), and J. F. Miskel on "The Chinese Opium Problem" (28: 3-14, 1973).

In *Medical History:* J. K. Crellin and J. R. Scott on "Pharmaceutical History . . . in the Wellcome Collections: III Fluid Medicine" (14: 132-153, 1970), and Sami Hamarneh on "Pharmacy in Medieval Islam and the History of Drug Addiction" (16: 226-237, 1972).

And, in *Bulletin of the History of Medicine,* J. Parascandola and R. Jasensky on "Origins of the Receptor Theory of Drug Action" (48: 199-220, 1974).

NAME INDEX

A

Abano, Pietro, 77
Abel, John Jacob, 173
Abdul-Chalig Achundow, 14, 80
Abu Al-Mina ibn Al-Attar, 78, 79
Abu Mansur Ali Haravi, 14, 80
Acosta, Cristovao, 89
Adam, 136
Adams, Francis, 12, 58, 70
Adlung, A., 12
Aesclepiades, 64
Aetius of Byzantium, 70
Agrippina, 65
Albertus Magnus, 86
Alexander the Great, 36
Alexander of Trales, 70
Al-Kindi, 76, 77
Alksnis, J., 14, 86
Allen, Edgar, 175
Alles, Gordon, 34, 176
Al-Razi, 77
Ammar, Sleim, 72, 73
Anderson, A. J. O., 54
Andre-Pontier, L., 12
Andrews, Edmund, 142
Andromachus, 66, 90
Anrep, Vasili K., 150
Apollodorus, 66
Apollonius Mus, 66
Arber, A. R., 13
Areius, 62
Aretaeus, 68
Aristotle, 59, 75
Arius (Bishop), 71
Arnold of Villanova, 86
Ashurpanipal, 38
Avenzoar, 79
Avicenna, 79, 85

B

Bach, J. S., 101
Badiano, Juan, 53
Balard, Antoine Jerome, 144
Bancroft, Wilder D., 126
Bankes, Rycharde, 90
Banting, Frederick G., 174
Barbour, Henry Gray, 163
Barger, George, 173, 177
Barrett, 12
Barton, William P. C., 132
Baumann, Eugen, 165, 174, 176
Beaumont, William, 179
Becker, Mrs. Hortense Koller, 152
Becquerel, Antoine Henri, 178
Beddoes, Thomas, 117
Behrend, H., 154
Bell, Charles, 122
Bell, J., 13
Benedicenti, A., 13
Berendes, J., 13
Bernard, Claude, 6, 22, 123, 125, 127, 130, 139, 172, 174, 178
Bert, Paul, 130
Berthollet, Claude Louis, 120
Best, Charles H., 174
Bigelow, Henry Jacob, 135
Binz, Karl, 165
Black, Joseph, 116
Blake, James, ix, 6, 123, 124, 127, 128, 139, 141, 144, 145, 148
Blegny, Nicholas de, 104
Bock, Jerome (Tragus), 91
Böhm, Rudolf, 148
Bontius, Jacobus, 180
Borgias, (the), 99
Borgognoni, Teodorico, 85
Boussel, P., 13
Bovet, Daniel, 187
Boyle, Robert, 101, 109, 110, 115
Bradley, Harold, 33
Breasted, James H., 48
Bretonneau, Pierre, 130
Bright, Richard, 107

Broussais, Francois Joseph, 130, 131
Brown, Alexander Crum, 22, 123, 145
Brown, William, 93
Browne, Eward Granville, 80
Brown-Sequard, Charles, 175
Brunfels, Otto, 91
Brunton, Thomas Lauder, 144, 145
Bucherl, W., 146
Buchheim, Rudolf, 137, 138, 146
Buckley, Eleanor, 146, 184
Bunge, George, 147
Burn, J. H., 7
Butler, Thomas, 150
Bynum, William F., 144

C

Cadwalader, Thomas, 185
Cahours, August Andre', 161
Calmette, Albert Leon Charles, 146
Cannon, Walter B., 34, 124, 178
Cartier, Jacques, 113
Cash, John Theodore, 144
Caspari, Charles, Jr., 29
Cavendish, Henry, 117
Caventou, Joseph B., 120
Cellini, Benvenuto, 96
Celsus, A. Cornelius, 66, 65
Cervantes, 101
Cervello, Vincenzo, 155, 175
Cesalpino, Andrea, 94
Chadwick, J., 28
Charles II, 109
Charles V., 95
Chen, Ko-Kui, 33
Chen, Li Shi, 32
Chisius, Carl, 114
Chopra, R. N., 15, 36, 37
Christison, Robert, 138, 183
Clark, Alfred Joseph, 6, 146
Clarke, William E., 133
Claudius, 65
Clouston, Thomas Smith, 154
Clover, Joseph Thomas, 142
Coindet, Jean Francois, 174
Coleman, Alfred, 162
Coleridge, Samuel Taylor, 182
Collip, James B., 174
Colton, Gradner Q., 133, 142
Constantine the Great, 69

Constantinus Africanus, 84
Cook, James, 114
Copernicus, Nicholas, 94
Cordus, Euricius, 91, 92
Cordus, Valerius, 7, 91, 94, 98, 132, 185
Corning, James Leonard, 153
Crandall, Lathan, 144
Crawford, Albert C., 173
Crookes, William, 130
Cruz, Martin de la, 53
Curie, Marie and Pierre, 178

D

Dale, Henry, 173, 175, 177
Dalton, John, 127, 141
Dam, Henrick, 182
Danilewski, Aleksander I., 182
Daremberg, C. V., 69
Darwin, Charles Robert, 111
Dastre, J. A. F., 143
Davis, Edgerton Y., Jr., 30
Davy, Humphrey, 118, 132
Demetisch, W., 14, 83
De Graaf, Regner, 115
De Quincy, Thomas, 182
De Rosemont, L. R., 13
Derosne, Louis Charles, 128
Dibble, C. E., 54
Dioscorides, 7, 28, 36, 60, 62, 73, 75, 80, 85, 93, 94, 135, 159, 177
Dodoens, Rembert, 90
Doisy, Edward, 175
Donders, Franciscus, 151
Dover, Thomas, 112
Dragendorff, G. J. N., 13
Dreser, Heinrich, 161, 162, 164
Duisburg, Carl, 159
Dumas, Jean Baptiste Andre, 121, 156
Dunstan, Wyndham Rowland, 144
Duran-Reynols, M. L., 103

E

Ebbell, B., 48
Ebers, Georg, 48
Efron, D. F., 15, 25
Ehrlich, Paul, 171, 172
Eichholtz, Fritz, 155
Eijkman, Christian, 180
Einhorn, Alfred, 152

Name Index

Elizabeth, my wife, viii
Elizabeth, Queen (1), 90
Ellis, Henry Havelock, 176
Elscholtz, Johann Sigmund, 108
Emmart, Emily W., 53
Empedocles, 59
Essakaly, Mohammed Eccherif, 73
Evans, Herbert McLean, 182
Eve, 136

F

Fabing, Howard, 43
Faraday, Michael, 127, 132
Fayrer, Joseph, 184
Featherstone, Robert, 150
Filehne, Wilhelm, 153, 160, 175
Fischer, Emil, 156, 157, 176
Fleming, Alexander, 182
Flourens, Pierre J. M., 135
Flückiger, F. A., 12
Fonseca, Olympia da, 106
Fontana, Felice, 115, 184
Fracastoro, Girolamo, 95
Fränkel, Sigmund, 143
Franklin, Benjamin, 185
Fraser, Thomas Richard, 6, 22, 123, 145, 184
Frazier, J. G., 23, 27
Freud, Sigmund, 150, 151, 152
Friedenwald, Harry, 45
Frobensius, J. A. S., 132
Fuchs, Leonhart, 91
Fulton, John F., 14
Funk, Casimir, 180
Fust, Johann, 88

G

Galen, 66, 67, 68, 72, 75, 84, 90
Galileo, 101, 114
Gamgee, Arthur, 144
Garcia de Huerta, 89
Garfield, Eugene, 187
Garrison, Fielding H., 31, 32, 44, 67, 75, 82, 85, 102
Garrod, Alfred Barin, 154
Gaskell, Walter, 172
Gay-Lussac, Joseph, 120
Geber, ibn Hajar, 73, 74, 75, 98
Geiger, Philipp Lounz, 121

Gerarde, John, 90
Gerhard, Wilhelm Wood, 131
Gerhardt, Charles Frederic, 161
Gesner, Conrad, 91
Gley, Eugene, 174
Glisson, Francis, 181
Glover, Robert Mortimer, 154
Goethe, Johann Wolfgang von, 137
Gomez, Bernardino Antonio, 106
Goodyear, John, 62
Gottlieb, Rudolph, 3
Graham, Thomas, 127
Grapow, Hermann, 47
Graves, Robert, 25, 27, 43, 65
Greenberg, Leon, 161
Greer, J., 13
Grew, Nehemiah, 111
Gross, Martin, 161
Guerney, B. G., 99
Guerra, Francisco, 25, 43, 53, 54, 55
Guibourt, G., 12
Guinter of Andernach, 68
Gunther, Robert, T., 62
Gutenberg, Johann, 88
Guthrie, Douglas, 27
Guthrie, Samuel, 135
Gutzeit, Conrad, 156
Guy de Chauliac, 86

H

Haggis, A. W., 103
Hahnemann, Christian F. S., 166
Hales, Stephen, 112, 127
Haller, Albrecht von, 112, 138
Halsted, William Stewart, 153
Haly Ben Abbas, 79
Hamarneh, Sami, 78
Hamilton, Alice, 184
Hammurabi, 39
Hanbury, D., 12
Hant-Ti, 31
Hare, H. A., 29
Harnack, E., 4
Harpenstreng, Henrick, 86
Harvey, William, 101, 108
Hassenfratz, Jean Henri, 117
Hata, Sahachiro, 172
Hauptmann, Alfred, 157
Hearst, Phoebe Apperson, 49

Heberden, William, 110
Heffter, Arthur, 176
Helvetius, J. C. A., 103
Henderson, V. E., 126
Henrici, A. A., 14, 83
Heraclitus, 59
Hernandez, Francisco, 54
Hess, Germain Henri, 121
Hickman, Henry Hill, 133
Hippocrates, 51, 75
Hirt, Ludwig, 184
Hoffman, Albert, 177
Hoffman, Friedrich, 111
Holmes, Oliver Wendell, 88, 131, 135
Holmstedt, Bo, 15, 103, 113, 157
Hooke, Robert, 111
Hopkins, Frederick Gowland, 181
Horn, Paul, 80
Huard, P., 31
Hunt, Reid, 173
Hunter, John, 106, 107

I

I-Yin, 32
Ibn Baitar, 80
Ibn Sarabionn (Serapion), 79
Ibn Sina (Avicenna), 79, 85
Isadore of Seville, 85
Ishaq, Honian (Johannitius), 80

J

Jackson, Charles T., 134
Jastrow, Morris, 38
Jenner, Edward, 107, 108
Jerome of Brunswick, 85
Jesus, 71
Jiminez-Porras, Jesus M., 184
Jobst and Hesse, 21
Johannitius, 80
Jolly, J., 80
Jones, W. H. S., 58
Julia Anicia, 62
Julian the Apostate, 66, 69

K

Karrer, Paul, 22
Kast, Alfred, 156, 159
Kastle, Jospeh Hoeing, 182
Kehoe, Robert A., 185

Kekule', Friedrich August, 8, 141
Keller, W., 147
Kettering, Charles Franklin, 185
Kitasato, Shibasaburo, 149, 172
Klebs, Arnold, 13, 89
Knoefel, Peter K., 114, 178
Knorr, Ludwig, 160
Kobert, Eduard Rudolf, 13, 80
Koch, Robert, 171
Kolbe, Adolph Wilhelm, 161
Koller, Carl, 150, 151, 152
Koppec, Richard, 147
Krantz, John Christian, Jr., 144, 162
Krateus, 61, 62
Kremers, E., 13
Kreig, Margaret, 15, 25, 26
Krukoff, B. A., 22

L

Labbe, L., 126
Laennec, Rene'-Theophile, 130
Lagrange, Joseph Louis, 117
Lal, K. K., 35
Lanman, C. R., 35
Landsteiner, Karl, 109
Langley, John Newport, 172
Lansing, Alfred, 15
Largus, Scribonius, 43, 68
Larkey, Sanford, 49, 90
Latham, Peter M., 57
Lavoisier, A. L., 8, 117, 120
La Wall, G. H., 13
LeClerc, Lucien, 80
Lemaire, Francois Jules, 158
Leonardo da Vinci, 99, 100
Leonicenus, 97
Leroux, 161
Lettsom, John, 131
Levy, A. G., 143
Levy, Martin, 76, 77, 78
Lewin, Louis, 4, 25, 176, 183
Liebig, Justus von, 122, 135, 154
Liebrich, Oscar, 154, 155
Lignamine, Filippo de, 89
Liljestrand, G., 15, 103, 113, 157
Lind, James, 114
Linne', Carl, 111
Lister, Joseph, 158, 171
Littre', Emile, 58

Locock, Charles, 154
Loevenhart, Arthur, 33, 153, 182
Long, Crawford, W., 133, 135
Long, Esmond R., 14
Louis XIV, 104, 109
Louis, Pierre Alexander, 130, 131
Lower, Richard, 109
Lucas, G. H. W., 126
Lucia, Salvatore, P., 23
Ludwig, Carl, 144, 148
Lunin, N., 181
Lutz, Henry, 49
Lydecker, Penny, viii

M

Macht, David I., 4
Magendie, Francois, 6, 122, 124, 127, 135, 138, 139
Magnus, Henrick Gustav, 117
Maimonides, Moses, 78, 79
Major, Ralph H., 14
Markham, Clements, 104
Marsh, David, 185
Marsh, James, 139, 183
Mattioli, Pietro, 94
Mayo, John, 110
McCollum, Elmer V., 181
McIntyre, A. R., 22
Meissner, K. F. W., 120
Mendeleyev, Dimitri, 128
Merck, Georg Franz, 121
Merck, George, 181
Merezhkowski, Dimitri, 28, 99
Merritt, Houston, 158
Mesue, 79, 80
Meyer, Hans Horst, 3, 148, 149
Ming Wong, 31
Minkowski, Oscar, 155, 174
Mitchell, Samuel Latham, 92
Mitchell, Silas Weir, 176
Mithridates, 62, 65
Modell, Walter, 15
Mohammed, 72, 73
Moliere, 101
Monardes, Nicolas, 89
Morpheus, 119
Morton, William T. G., 133, 134, 135
Mravlag, Victor, 152
Muehlbacher, C. A., 150

Müller, G., 51
Murray, George R., 174
Murrell, William, 144

N

Naaman, 44
Needham, Joseph, 31
Neimann, Albert 121
Nestorius, 71
Neumann, John von, 124
Newcomen, Thomas, 117
Newton, Isaac, 101, 111
Nikander, 65, 66, 183
Nileus, 66
Nineb, 39
Noah, 24, 42
Nunnely, Thomas, 126

O

Oldenberg, Henry, 109
Oliver, George, 173
Oliver, Thomas, 184
Olivera, H., 43, 55
Olmsted, J. M. D., 122, 124
O'Malley, Charles D., 95
Omrane, Isaac ibn, 72
Orfila, Mathien Joseph, 138, 183
Oribasius, 66, 69
Ortoff of Wurzburg, 89
Osler, William, 2, 101, 119
Overton, Charles Ernest, 149
Oviedo, F. de, 89

P

Page, Irvine H., 175
Paracelsus, 75, 97, 98
Pare', Ambrose, 97
Parkinson, John, 90
Pasteur, Louis, 158
Pauling, Linus, 150
Paul of Aegina, 12, 70
Pavlov, Ivan, 179
Pechey, John, 102
Pelletier, Pierre Joseph, 120, 121
Penfield, Wilder, 57
Percival, Thomas, 107
Pereirra, Jonathon, 137
Perkin, William Henry, 158
Peters, H., 13

Phipps, James, 108
Pinel, Phillippe, 131
Piria, Rafael, 158, 161
Pirigoff, Nikolai I., 135
Piso, Wilhelm, 103
Platearius, Mathaeus, 85
Pliny, 66, 68, 102
Poiseuille, Jean Marie, 127
Pope, Alexander, 3
Pott, Percival, 112
Priestley, Joseph, 116
Purkyne, Jan Evangelista, 137
Putnam, Tracy Jackson, 157

R

Ramazzini, Bernadino, 184
Rauwolf, Leonard, 177
Read, Bernard, 34
Redard, P., 148
Redwood, T., 13
Reichert, Edward, 184
Reichstein, Tadeus, 180
Reisner, George, 49
Rembrandt, 101
Rhazes (Al-Razi), 79
Richardson, Benjamin Ward, 143, 149
Richter, G. H., 126
Ricord, Philippe, 131
Robiquet, Pierre Jean, 121
Roelants, Joachim, 95
Roentgen, Wilhelm Conrad, 178, 179
Roger of Palermo, 85
Romanell, Patrick, ix
Ronsaeus, Baldiunus, 113, 180
Rosarius, Johann, 69
Rosen, George, 98
Ruelle, Jean, 94
Rufus of Ephesus, 68
Runge, Friedlieb Ferdinand, 121, 158
Rusby, H. H., 29

S

Sahli, Hermann, 165
Samson, 25
Santorio, Santorio, 114
Saunders, J. B. deC. M., 57
Scheele, Carl Wilhelm, 112
Schelenz, H., 13

Schipperges, H., 84
Schleich, Carl Ludwig, 153
Schmidt, C. F., 34
Schmiedeberg, Oswald, 123, 146, 148, 155, 156, 161
Schoffer, Peter, 88
Schutte, D., 181
Schwann, Theodore, 182
Seguin, Armand, 120
Selkirk, Alex. (Robinson Crusoe), 112
Semmelweis, Ignaz Philipp, 131
Serapion, 79
Sertürner, Friedrick W. A., 8, 119
Shakespeare, William, 71, 82, 101
Sharpey, William, 127
Sharpey-Schäffer, Edward, 173
Shen-Nung, 31
Shuster, Louis, 15
Sigerist, Henry E., 98
Siggel, Alfred, 74
Silverman, Milton, vi, ix, 15, 157, 159, 161, 171
Simpson, James Young, 135
Singer, Charles, 13, 61, 62, 99
Sloane, Hans, 113
Smith, Ashbel, ix
Smith, Edgar Fahs, 117
Smith, Paul K., 160
Snow, John, 136, 142, 143
Socrates, 121
Soleiman, Isaac ibn, 72
Soranus of Ephesus, 68
Souberain, Eugene, 135
Spaulding, Lyman, 92
Squibb, Edward R., 141
St. Martin, Alexis, 179
Stahl, George Ernest, 116
Steenbock, Harry, 181
Steinschneider, Moritz, 80
Steuer, Robert, 57
Stoll, Arthur, 177
Stone, Edward, 161
Störck, Anton, 115
Strecher, Paul G., 63
Stricker, Solomon, 161
Sutherland, Earl W., 187
Sydenham, Thomas, 104
Szent-Gyorgi, Albert, 180

T

Tainter, Maurice, 161
Takaki, Kanehiro, 180
Takamine, Jokichi, 173
Talbor, Robert, 104
Taylor, Frances Long, 133
Temkin, Owsei, 98
Thales, 59
Theophrastus, 28, 60, 68
Thomas, Charles C., 14
Thompson, Benjamin (Rumford), 117
Thompson, C. J. S., 13
Thompson, R. C., 38
Tigerstedt, Robert Adolf, 175
Torti, Francesco, 104
Tragus (Jerome Bock), 91
Trevan, J. W., 6, 8, 123
Turner, M., 132
Turner, William, 90
Tyndall, John, 182

U

Urdang, G., 12, 13

V

Valentine, Basil, 98
Valle, Jose A. do, 106
Van der Hoeven, C. P., 12
Van Helmont, Jean Baptiste, 116
Vassali, Guilio, 175
Vegetius, Publius, 70
Veith, Ilza, 31
Ventris, M. 28
Vesalius, Andreas, 94, 95, 96, 97
Viatique, 72
Virgil, viii
Vitruvius, 181
Von Behring, Emil Adolf, 148, 171
Von Euler, Ulf Svante, 187

Von Grot, R., 14
Von Henria, Alfred, 86
Von Kalb, Johann, 89
Von Mering, Josef, 123, 155, 156, 159, 174
Von Nencki, Marcel, 6, 123, 165

W

Waldie, James, 135
Waring, E. J., 12
Warren, C. P. W., 28
Warren, John Collins, 133
Wasson, Gordon, 24, 43
Waters, Ralph, 133
Watson, Gilbert, 65, 66
Watt, James, 117
Weber, E. H., 137
Wellman, Max, 94
Wells, Horace, 133
Wepfer, Johannes, 115
Whitney, W. D., 35
Wiener, Norbert, 124, 179
Williams, Robert R., 180, 181
Willis, Thomas, 110
Willstätter, Richard, 153
Winterstein, O., 22
Withering, William, 106, 107
Wöhler, Friedrich, 121, 122
Wood, Alexander, 142
Woodall, John, 113
Wootton, A. C., 13
Wren, Christopher, 109

Z

Zad el Moucafir, 72
Zahagun, Bernadino, 53, 54
Zainer, 89
Zilbourg, Gregory, 98
Zimmer, Henry A., 36

SUBJECT INDEX

A

Abbessiche era of Muslim medicine, 73
Absorption and excretion of drugs, 123
Acadamia dei Lincei, 109
Academie des Sciences (Paris), 109
Accessory food factors, 181
Acetaldehyde, 155
Acetone, 110
Acetphenetidin, 156, 159, 160
Acetyl salicylic acid (aspirin), 159, 161
Acetylation, 159
Aconite (wolfsbane), 27, 28, 115, 120
Aconitine, 120
Acupuncture, 32, 188
Addiction, 150
Adenosine monophosphate, cyclic (AMP), 187
Adrenal glands, 173
Adrenalin, 173
Adulteration of drugs, 7, 61
Agranulocytosis, 160
Agricultural pharmacology, 129
Agriculture, development of, 38
Alchemy, 73, 98
Alcohol (ethanol), 73, 92, 138, 149, 155
Alcoholic beverages, abuse of, 183
Alcoholism, 131
Alcohols, straight-chained, 143
Alexipharmaca, of Nicander, 65
Alkaloid, naming of, 120
Aliphatic compounds, 149
Alkyl compounds, 143
Allgemeines Krankenhaus, 132
Almonds, 122
Alum as styptic, 98
Amanita muscaria, 24, 147
American pharmacopeias, 92, 93
Amidopyrine, 160, 175
Amines, structure and action of, 173
Amino-benzoic acid, 152
Ammonia, 98
Ammonium cyanate, 122

Amoebic dysentery, 103
Amphetamines, 173, 176
Amygdalin, 122
Amyl nitrite, 144
Amylene hydrate, 155, 156
Ancient Physician's Legacy (Dover's), 112
Anesthesia, 132, 135, 141
Anesthesia, local, 143
Anesthesia, theories of, 124, 125, 149, 150
Anesthetic agents, action of, 124, 149
Anesthetic sponge, 86
Anesthetic substances, 136
Angina pectoris, 144
Angiotensin, 107
Aniline, 121, 158
Annotationes in Pedacii Dioscorides of Valerius Cordus, 91, 92
Anodynes, ancient, 21
Anoxemia, 130
Anterior pituitary extracts, 175
Anthelmintics, 138, 148
Anthracene, 121
Antibiotics, 170, 182
Antidiarrheal drugs, 19
Antidotarium of Nicolas of Salerno, 85
Antidote, universal, 65
Antidotes of Galen, 66
Antidotes of poisons, 138
Antigens, 163
Antihemorrhagic factor, 182
Antihistaminics, 187
Antimony salts, 98, 148
Antipyretic analgesics, 156, 158, 163, 165
Antipyrine, 153, 160, 175
Antiseptics, 132, 158
Antivenom serum, 146, 184
Apothecaries, 102
Aqrabadhin of Al-Kindi, 76, 77
Aqua regia, 73
Arabic language, 71

199

Arabic Medicine by Browne, 80
Arbor vitae (*Thuja occidentalis*), 113
Archives für Experimentellen Pathologie und Pharmakologie, 148, 187
Aromatic organic compounds, 141
Arrow poisons, 115
Arsenic trioxide, 75, 99, 171, 183
Arsenical compounds, 171
Arsenical poisoning, 183
Arsenical salts, 99, 138, 148
Arthritis, 22, 158, 160
Artificiosis extractionibus of Valerius Cordus, 92
Artzneibuch of Ortoff, 89
Arzneimittelsynthese of S. Fränkel, 143
Ascorbic acid, 180
Asphyxia, 124, 125, 135
Aspirin (acetylsalicylic acid), 160, 162
Aspirin, mechanism of action of, 162, 164
Assyrian medical texts, 38
Asthma, 33, 176
Astringent antiseptic, garlic as, 52
Astrology in relation to drug use, 41, 73
Atomic theory, 141
Atomic weight, 128
"Atoxyl" of R. Koch, 171
Atropine, 121, 126, 143, 145, 147, 153, 173
Aurum potible (colloidal gold), 74
Autonomic drugs, 170
Autonomic nervous system, 145, 172
"Avertin," 155
Aviation, 130
Avium praecipuarum, 90
Aztec drugs, 54
Aztec herbals, 53

B

Bacteria, 158
Badianus Codex, 53
Baghdad, 72
Balsam of Tolu, 104
Banda Island, 102
Barbital, 176
Barbituric acid, 157, 176
Barium carbonate (Witherite), 106
Barium salts, 148, 178
Bark, The, 103

Baroque culture, 100, 101
Basel, 97
Bayer aspirin, legal aspects of 162
Beers, 23, 39, 41
Belladonna, 121, 173
"Bends" (caisson disease), 130
Bengala beans, 103
Benzene, 136
Benzoic acid, 147, 153
Beri-beri, 180
Berlin medical papyrus, 47
Bhang, 75
Bhuddism, 32
Bile, necessary for digestion of fat, 112
Binary notation of old Egyptians, 46
Biochemorphology, 144, 145, 155
Biogenic amines, 187
Biological standardization of drugs, 7
Bismuth ointments, 112
Bismuth salts, 178
Blatta bizantina (dried cockroach?), 102
Bleeding, treatment by, 59, 131
Blood, analysis of, 110
Blood pressure, 127
Blood sugar, 174
Blood transfusions, 109
Book of the Natures of All Wines, 90
Borax, 75
Borgias, 99, 183
Botanologicon of E. Cordus, 91
Brazilian medicinal plants, 105, 106
Breslau, 139
British Association for the Advancement of Science, 128
Brombenzen-xylene method for specific gravity, 164
Bromide ion, 154
Bromoform, 136
Brucine, 120, 145
"Bufferin," 162
Bufotonin, 34
Bureaucratic control of drugs, 170, 185
Byzantine compilers, 69

C

Caffeine, 120
Caisson disease ("bends"), 130
Calabar bean, 105, 139, 145
Calcium chloride, 132

Subject Index

Calcium ions, 149
California Academy of Sciences, 129
Calomel, 144
Camphor, 137
Cannabis indica, 35, 41, 42, 185
Canon of Avicenna, 79
Carbamic acid, 156
Carbolic Acid, 158
Carbon cycle between plants and animals, 122
Carbon bisulfide (or disulfide), 129, 136
Carbon-dioxide (fixed air), 116, 133, 136
Carbon monoxide, 97, 124, 125
Cardomomum malabaricum, 103
Carminatives, 52, 101
Cascara sagrada, 19
Cassine, 102
Castor oil, 52
Cataract operation, anesthesia in, 151
Catecholamines, 173, 177
Cathartics, 138
Cautery, 76
Celluloses, 177
Central nervous system depressants, 153
Central nervous system drugs, 170
Cerebellar cells, 137
Ceylon, 102
Charaka Samahita, 35
Chemical analysis, 139
Chemical analysis, techniques of, 119
Chemical warfare, 184
Chemistry, empirical, 98
Chemotherapy, 170
Chemotherapy of syphilis, 172
China root, 95
Chinese drug lore, 31
Chinese drugs, list of, 33
Chinese materia medica, 33, 188
Chinese pharmacies, 33
Chloral hydrate, 122, 154, 175
Chloralformamide, 155
Chlorbutanol, 155
Chloretone, 155
Chlorine bleach, 120
Chlorine gas, 131
Chloroform, 122, 125, 135, 137, 138, 142, 154
Chlorophylls, 177

Chocolate, 105
Cholera, 89, 136
Choline derivatives, 173
Ciliary motion, drug action on, 137
Cinchona bark, 103, 120
Cinchona in Java, 104
Cinnamon, 102
Cinnebar (mercuric sulfide), 75
Circulation time, 127
Circumcision, 44
Citric and organic acids, 112
Classification of drugs by Geber, 75
Classification of plants, 60
Clathrate crystal theory of anesthesia, 150
Claviceps purpurea, 111
Cloud berries (Rubus) for scurvy, 114
Cloves, 102
Clyster, 142
Cnidian medicine, 67
Cnidos, 57
Coagulation, reversible in anesthesia, 126
Cobra venom, 146
Cocaine, 21, 56, 121, 150, 153,
Coca leaves, 21, 56, 121
Cacao, 105
Codex medicamentarius (French pharmacopeia), 92
Codeine, 121, 145
Cod-liver oil, 107, 181
Codoba, 79
Coffee, 105, 120
Colchicine, 120, 121
Colchicum for gout, 121
Collyrium of Abu Mohammed, 77
Cologuios dos simples by Garcia de Huerta, 89
Columbo wood (cinnamon?), 102
Compositiones medicorum by Scrib. Largus, 68
Computers, 179
Condiments, 101
Conditioned reflexes, 179
Coniine, 121, 139, 145
Co-ordinated research endeavor, 9
Copper salts, 75, 99
Cornplasters, 159
Cosmetic recipes, Egyptian, 48, 51

Council of Nicea, 71
Cowpox vaccine, 108
Croccus (Colchicum), 120, 121
Crocus metallorum (antimony salts), 109
Croton oil, 148
Cruydesboek by Dodoena, 90
Curare, 22, 105, 124, 125
Curare action of quaternary ammonium, 145
Currus triumphalis antimonii, 98
Cybernetics, 179
Cyclamen, 27

D

Damascus, 73
Danske Laegebog (herb remedies), 86
Datura stramonium, 121
Decamethonium compounds, 22
De Motu Cordis by William Harvey, 108
Dental extraction, 134
Dephlogisticated air (oxygen), 116
De Plantis by Cesalpinus, 94
De Revolutionibus by Copernicus, 94
De Simplicibus by Galen, 66
Desert sores, 44
Detoxification, 147
Diabetes mellitus, 155, 174
Diacetyl morphine (heroine), 164
Diagnosis by inspection, 38
Diagnostic drugs, 170
Diarrhea, barks for, 19
Diet, 18, 58, 79
Diethyl-malonyl-urea (barbital), 156
Digitalis glucosides, 148
Digitalis purpurea, 106, 107
"Dilantin," 158
Diphenyl hydantoin, 157
Diphtheria antitoxin, 149
Disease, Classic Descriptions of, 14
Disinfectant, 158
Dispensatorium of Valerius Cordus, 92
Distillation, 73
Diuretic action of digitalis, 144
Diuretics, Egyptian, 52
Dos Libros of Monardes, 89
Dose-effect relations, 6, 123
Dover's powder, 112

"Dragon's blood," 53
Dropsy, 106
Drug abuse, social control of, 183
Drug action, undesired, 4
Drug compendia, Muslim, 76
Drug development in the Renaissance, 88
Drug evaluation, 9
Drug gardens, 83
Drug industry, 141
Drug innovations by Muslims, 71
Drug, intensity of action of, 169
Drug, mechanism of action of, 123
Drug name synonyms, 77
Drug, relation of structure to action, 123
Drug, standardization, 7
Drug standards, 93
Drug effects on particular organs, 115
Drug trade, 89, 102
Drug use, empirical, 19, 30
Drugs (Life Science Library), 15
Drugs, absorption & distribution of, 122, 123
Drugs, diagnostic, 170
Drugs, Egyptian, 51, 52
Drugs, historical account of, 12
Drugs, homeopathic, 168
Drugs, identification of, 76
Drugs in 17th & 18th centuries, 101
Drugs in Medieval Europe, 82
Drugs, no miracle, 17
Drugs of India, 15, 36, 37, 89
Drugs, site of action of, 123
Drugs, sleep producing, 153
Drugs, social control of, 24, 182
Drugs, Sumerian, 38
Drugs, sustained release of, 165
Drugs, systematic experiments with, 115
Dutch drug trade, 102
Dysmenorrhea, 154

E

East India Company, 102
Ebers medical papyrus, 6, 48
Ecological effects of chemicals, 170
Edessa, 72
Edinburgh, 107, 123, 136, 139, 145, 146
Edwin Smith surgical papyrus, 47, 48

Subject Index

Egyptian binary notation, 46
Egyptian carminatives, 52
Egyptian drug codification, 45
Egyptian drug formularies, 48, 49
Egyptian drug lists, 51
Egyptian hieroglyphs, 47
Egyptian medical papyri, 47, 50
Egyptian pharmacists, 46
Egyptian principle of putrefaction, 51
Elements (water, fire, air, water), 59
Elements, chemical isolation of, 118, 122
Elixir of life, 74
Elizabeth, New Jersey, 152
Emetics, 131
Emetics, prehistoric, 19, 20
Emetine, 21, 103, 122
Emodin, 148
Empirical drug use, 19
Endocrine drugs, 170
Endocrinology, 168
English herbals, 90
Enzyme action, reversible, 182
Enzymes, 168, 182
Enzyme mediation in drug action, 170
Ephedra vulgaris, 33
Ephedrine, 33, 176
Epilepsy, 154, 157
Epinephrine, 173, 176
Epinephrine release, 143, 179
Epsom salts (Magnesium sulfate), 111
Ergot, 75, 111, 177
Ergot alkaloids, 177
Ergotism, 83, 111
Erman medical papyrus, 49
Erythrol tetranitrate, 144
Estrogen, 175
Ethanol, 155
Ether, 92, 98, 125, 132, 135, 137, 141
Ether frolics, 133
Ethnopharmacologic Search, 15
Ethyl bromide, 136
Ethyl chloride, 135
Ethyl nitrate, 135
Ethylene, 136
Etiology, Egyptian *(whd)*, 51
Evaluation of drugs, 9
Exploratory voyages, 89

F

Fabrica Corporis humani (Vesalius), 94
Feed-back control mechanisms, 178
Fermentation, lactic, 182
Fever-Bark Tree (Duran-Reynolds), 103
Fevers, 163
Filtration, 73
Folk-remedies, 137
Food & Drug Administration of USA, 7, 186
Food poisoning, 99
Foods, classification of, 122
Foods, qualities of, 59, 60, 69
Formulaire by Magendie, 123
Formularies, Egyptian, 48, 49
Formulary of Al-Kindi, 77
Fox-glove, 106
Franco-Prussian War, 146
Fuliginous vapors of Galen, 117
Fundamentalism, 136
Fungi, 182

G

Galenicals, 66
Galen's *Antidotes*, 66
Galen's *De Compositione*, 77
Galen's *De Simplicibus*, 66
Galen's physiological schema, 67
Gandisapor, 72
Ganglionic synapses, 172
Garlic, 36, 52
Gart der Gesundheit, 89
Gaultheria, oil of (wintergreen), 161
Geology, 129
Germ theory, 131
German herbalists, 91
German pharmacology, 137, 146
German precisionists, 16
Ginseng, 27, 102
Glycine, 147, 163
Glycogenic function of liver, 124, 174
Glycuronic acid, 148, 155, 163
Goiter, 174
Gold, colloidal, 74
Gold rush to California, 129
Gout, 154
Graeco-Roman medicine, 57
Green Medicine by M. Kreig, 15

H

Guaiacum, 96
Guild of St. Luke, 100

H

Hallucinating drugs, 176, 177
Hallucinating drugs from Mexico, 55
Halogenated hydrocarbons, 136, 143
Hammurabi, Code of, 39
Hashish, 42, 183
Healing power of nature, 58
Hearst Medical Papyrus, 49
Hebrew medicine, 44
Hellebore (veratrum), 63, 120
Hemlock (conium vespa), 115
Hemoconcentration, 163
Hemodynameter, 124
Hemp (cannabis indica), 41, 42
Henbane (hyoscyamus), 121
Hepato-toxicity, 143
Herb distillates, 86
Herb gardens, 111
Herbal, Gerarde's, 90
Herbals, catalogue of early, 89
Herbals, English, 90
Herbals, lists of, 13
Herbarium vivae eicones by Brunfels, 91
Herbarius Apuleius, 89
Herbarius Moguntunus, 88
Herbs, 87
Heroin, addiction, 165
Hiera, purgative of Rufus, 68
Hieratic writing, 47
Hieroglyphs, 47
Hindu drugs, 35, 37
Hippocratic physicians, 58
Hippocratic writings, 58
Hippuric acid, 122, 147
Histamine, 163
Historia plantarum by Gesner, 91
Historia stirpium by Fuchs, 91
Historical account of drugs, 12
Histories of pharmacy, 12, 13
Hoffman's Anodyne (tincture of opium), 112
Homeopathic drugs, 168
Homeostasis, 124, 178
Homicidal use of poisons, 99, 183
Honey, 52

Hortus Sanitatis, 89
Horus Eye, 51
Humoral pathology, 59
Humors, four, 59, 60
Hydantoins, 157
Hydrocarbons, 143
Hydropyrimidines, 157
Hydroquinone, 122
Hydrogen sulfide, 112
Hydrotherapy, 64
Hygienic laws of Hebrews, 45
Hyoscyamine, 121
Hyoscyamus, 35, 85, 115
Hypodermic syringe, 142

I

Ice-cover theory of anesthesia, 150
I. G. Farbinindustrie, 159
Ilex, species of, 105
Illustrations of plant drugs, 61
Immune bodies, 108
Immunology, 108
Immune preparations, 149
Incunabula, 88
Identification of drugs, 61
India, list of drugs from, 36, 37
India, plant drugs of, 36, 37, 89
Indole derivatives, 42
Industrial toxicology, 184
Infiltration anesthesia, 153
Inoculation for small pox, 107
Insomnia, 154
Institute for Scientific Information, 187
Insulin, 174
Internal secretion, 174
Internal steady state, 178
International Congress of Pharmacology, vii
Intravenous injection of drugs, 108, 109
Iodine, 174
Iodoform, 154
Ipecac, 103, 106, 122
Irish leech-books, 86
Iron salts, 99
Isomorphism, 129

J

Jami (Muslim materia medica), 80
Java, 104

Subject Index

Jewish medicine, 39, 45
Julia Anicia manuscript of Dioscorides, 62, 93
Juniper berries, 52

K
Kahun medical papyrus, 47
Kairouan, 72
Kava, 25
Kew Garden, 111
Kitab-As-sumum book of poisons, 74
Kitab fi-kimiya of Al-Kindi, 76
Kosher fit for food, 45
Knossus, 28
Kos, 57

L
LSD, 177
Lanolin, 155
Laurus camphora, 137
Lead acetate, 98
Lead poisoning, 185
Lead salts, 138
Lecons sur les Anesthesiques (Bernard), 124
Lecons sur les effets des substances toxique, 124
Le grand herbier, 89
Lehrbuch der Arzneimittellehre (Buchheim), 138
Lemons, 113, 180
Leprosy, 39
Letheon: Cadenced Story of Anesthesia, 20
Library of Assyrian clay tablets, 38
Lime juice, 114, 180
Linear B tablets, 28
Lithium bromide, 154
Living material, organizational levels of, 5
Local anesthesia, 143, 150
London pharmacopeias, 113
London medical papyrus, 49, 50
"Luminal," 157, 176
Lung disorders of miners, 98
Lysergic acid, 177

M
Maeyer-Overton theory of narcosis, 150

Magic in a Bottle (Silverman), 15, 157, 159, 171
Magical remedies condemned, 97
Ma Huang, 33
Malabar nuts, 103
Malaria, 104
Male fern (Felix-mas), 148
Mandragora, 27, 63, 68, 85
Marijuana, 42
Marsh test for arsenic, 139
Massachusetts General Hospital, 133, 134
Massage, 64
Materia medica, 146
Materia medica of Dioscorides, 61
Materia peccans, 51
Mayan prescriptions, 55
Mead (beverage), 83
Measurement of drugs (Egyptian), 46
Measurement of time, 38, 39
Medical jurisprudence, 183
Medical practice, Summerian specialization in, 39
Merck Index, 7, 63, 93
Merck Manual, 6, 64
Merck Veterinary Manual, 64
Mercurial ointments, 86, 96
Mercurous chloride, 144
Mercury, specific for syphilis, 99
Mescaline, 176
Metals, hierarchy of, 74
Meterology, 129
Methane, 136
Methyl alcohol, 121, 156
Methyl salicylate, 160
Micky Finns, 155
Micro-organisms as causes of disease, 171
Mid-American medicine, 53
Milieu interieur, 124
Milk, 52
Milk sugar, 166
Mineral waters, 106, 129
Mineral drugs of Geber, 75
Mithqal, 77
Mithridatium and Theriac, attack upon, 110
Mithridatum, 62
Molucca, 102

Molucca nuts (cloves?), 102, 103
Monasteries, 83
Monte Cassino, 89
Montpelier, 72, 86
Moon, significance of, 40
Morphine, 8, 119, 126, 142, 145, 150, 162
Mount St. Helena, 130
Moxa, 32
Muriatic acid, 98
Muscarine, 147
Mushrooms, hallucinating, 24, 43, 183
Muslim drug innovations, 71
Muslim formularies, 77
Muslim hospitals, 76
Muslim synonym drug lists, 77, 78
Muslim materia medica, 80
Mustard gas (dichlor-ethyl-sulfide), 185, 187
Mu'tazilite sect, 76
Myths, 27

N
Narceine, 121
Narcosis, 126
Narcosis, theory of, 149
Narcotine, 121
National Standard Dispensatory, 29
Naturopaths, 168
Nei-Ching, 31
Nerve gas (Dichlor-diethylamide), 187
Nerves, spinal, function of, 122
Nestorian sect of Arians, 72
Neue Kreuter Buch of Jerome Bock, 91
Nevada Great Basin, 129
New Herbal of Turner, 90
Nicotine, 145, 172
Nitrates, organic, 144
Nitric acid, 73
Nitro-aer (oxygen), 110
Nitrogen, 116, 130
Nitrogen cycle between plants & animals, 122
Nitroglycerine, 144
Nitrous oxide, 116, 118, 132, 135, 142
Norepinephrine, 173
Novocaine, 152
Nuovo Receptario, 92
Nuremberg Dispensatorium, 92

Nutmeg, 25, 102
Nux vomica, 20, 120, 122, 139

O
Ointments, 52
Oleum dulce vitrioli (ether), 92
Oliliuqui, hallucinating plant, 55, 177
Ommeiadic era of Muslim medicine, 73
Opium, 43, 68, 85, 109, 119, 120, 121, 137, 138,
Oranges, 113, 180
Organological arrangement, 138
Orgnaometallic compounds, 170
Organizational levels of living material, 5, 9, 138, 168
Ovarian hormone, 175
Ovulation, 175
Oxygen search for, 110
Oxygen toxicity, 130

P
Pacific Medical & Surgical Journal, 129
Pain, 20, 162, 163
p-amino phenol, 159
Panaquilon, 102
Panax ginseng, 102
Pancreas, 155
Pancreatic juice, digestive function of, 174
Papaver somniferum, 43
Papaverine, 121
Papyri, old Egyptian medical, 46
Paraldehyde, 155, 175
Parasympathetic nervous system, 145, 172
Parathormone, 174
Parathyroid glands, 174
Parisian determinists, 16
Partition co-efficient, 149
Pathology, humoral, 59
Pathology, Readings in by Esmond Long, 14
Pen T'sao, 31, 188
Penicillium, 182
Pepsin, 182
Perfusion of kidneys, 147
Pergamon, 66, 69
Periodic Table, 128
Persian medicine, 39, 72

Subject Index

Peruvian balsam, 103
Peruvian Bark (cinchona), 103
Pest control, 130, 187
Peyotl cactus, 55, 176
Pharmaceutica rationalis by Willis, 110
Pharmaceutical preparations of Muslims, 73
Pharmacists, Egyptian, 46
Pharmacologists, library & laboratory, 187
Pharmacology, applications of, 5
Pharmacology, definition of, 3
Pharmacology, University of Dorpat, 14
Pharmacology, modern, 167
Pharmacology, molecular, 141
Pharmacology, problems of, 6, 123, 167
Pharmacology, Readings in (Holmstedt), 15
Pharmacology, transition to 20th cent., 170
Pharmacopeia (Cordus), 92, 185
Pharmacopeia Londinensis, 92, 116, 185
Pharmacopeias, 13, 64, 92, 93, 116, 185
Pharmacopeias, American, 93, 94, 113, 185
"Phenacetin," 156, 159
Phenobarbital, 157
Phenol, 121
Phenyl butazone, 160
Phenyl-ethyl-malonyl-urea, 157
Phenyl salicylate (salol), 165
Philosopher's stone, 73
Phlogiston theory, 116
Phloridzin, 155
Phosphorus, 148
Phylloxera, 129
Physic gardens, 111
Physician's Desk Reference, 7
Physiological schema of Galen, 67
Physiology, history of, 14
Physostigma venenosum, 139
Physostigmine, 21, 145, 173
Picrotoxin, 154
"Pill," The, 175
Pilocarpine, 173
Pilocarpus, 105
Pine oils, 114
Pituitary body, 175
Placebo effect, 58

Plant drugs of India, 35
Plant remedies of Central America, 54, 96
Plantas Medicinais do Brazil (Gomez), 106
Platinum salts, 148
Pneumatic Institute (Beddoes), 117
Pneumonia, 131
Poisoning, homocidal, 99
Poisons and poisoning, 4, 62, 65
Poisons, book on, by Geber, 74
Poisonous, 98
Pollution of Boston Harbor, 112
Polypeptides, 175
Pomegranate, 78
Poppy, 43
Portugese drug trade, 102
Posterior pituitary extracts, 175
Potassium bromide, 153
Potassium sulfate, 98
Prague, 137
Prairie du Chien, Wisconsin, 179
Prehistoric empirical drug lore, 17
Prescription formularies, 76
Prescriptions in Ebers papyrus, 48
Principia (Newton), 111
Printing, development of, 88
Procaine, 153
Prognosis by augury, 38
Prolegomenon to Current Pharmacology, 9
Prostaglandins, 187
Proteins in anesthesia, 150
Protopharmacology, 17, 30
Psilocybin, 177
Psychiatry, 131
Psychoactive drugs, 170
Puerperal fever, 131
Pulmonaria, 27
Purgative drugs, Muslim classification, 80
Purgative drugs, prehistoric, 19
Purgatives, 131
Purgatives, Egyptian, 51
Purging, treatment by, 19, 51, 59
Purines, 156
"Pyramidon," 160
Pyrazole, 160
Pyrrole, 121

Q

Quackery, 60
Qualities of elements, 59
Qualities of foods, 59, 60, 69
Qualities of humors, 59
Quantitative chemical procedures, 8
Quantitative methods, 114, 118, 139, 140
Quaternary ammonium bases, 145
Quicksilver, 73, 75
Quinine, 21, 120, 158, 175
Quinoline, 158

R

Radiant energy, 178
Radiation physics, 168
Radioactive diagnostic drugs, 170
Radio-opaque diagnostic agents, 170, 179
Radix Chinae (China Root), 96
Rational use of drugs, 9, 10
Rauwolfia, 36, 177
Rectal anesthesia, 155
Redox potential, 180
Reformation, 100
Regimen Sanitatis, 84
Rejuvenation, 175
Remedi Anglois (de Blegny), 104
Renaissance, 100
Renin, 107, 175
Reserpine, 36, 177
Resins, 177
Respiratory gases, 117
De Revolutionibus (Copernicus), 94
Rheumatic fever, 161
Rheumatism, 22, 158, 160
Rhubarb, 79
Rice, polished, 180
Richardson's principle, 143, 153
Rickets, 181
Romance of Leonardo, 99
Roentgen-ray visualization, 178
Royal Botanical Gardens, Kew, 111
Royal College of Physicians, 92
Royal Society of London, 109
Ro, hieroglyph for mouthful, 46
Russian folk medicine, 86
Rye, smutty, 83

S

S.S.S., "blood purifier," 96
Sacramento, 129
Saffron, 27
Salap mucilage, 102, 103
Salerno, 72, 83, 84
Salicin, 158, 160
Salicylates, 161
Salicylic acid, 158, 160
Salol, 165
Salt, 18
Salts, inorganic, 128, 138
Salts of heavy metals, 138
Salts of rare earths, 130
"Salvarsan," 171, 176
Salzburg, 97
Samme de shinda sleeping potion, 45
San Francisco, vii
Sarsaparilla, 96, 114
Sassafras, 96, 114
Schizophrenia, 133
Schmiedeberg's Archives, 148
Scurvy, 113, 180
Seaweed for goiter, 85, 174
Seidlitz Powders, 111
Self-experimentation with drugs, 137
Serotonin, 175
Sevilla, 89
Sex hormones, 175
Side-chain theory of Ehrlich, 172
Signatures, doctrine of, 26, 33
Site of action of drugs, 6
Skeptical Chemist (Boyle), 110
Sleep-producing drugs, 175
Smallpox, 107
Smilax, 96
Snake-root (Rauwolfia), 36, 177
Snake venoms, 115, 184
Social control of drugs, 24
Social dangers of drugs, 182
Sodium salicylate, 161
Soporifics, 156
Sour oil of vitriol (sulfuric acid), 73, 92
Specialization in Sumerian medicine, 39
Specificum purgans Paracelsi (K_2SO_4), 98
Spectroscope, 130
Spice trade, 89

Subject Index

Spices, 101
Spirochaetes, 171
Spongia somnifera, 85
St. Anthony's Fire, 83
St. Bartholomew's Hospital, 144
St. Ignatius bean (Strychnos), 122
St. Louis, 129
Staining of cells and bacteria, 172
Standardization of drugs, 7, 149
Standardized drugs, 141
Statistical technique, 131
Steam engine, 117
Sterols, 175
Stethescopes, 130
Stirpium historiae of Dodoens, 91
Stonehenge, 41
Stomach, movement and secretions of, 179
Stramonium, 115
Strassburg, 147
Strophanthus, 20, 105, 145
Structure-action relations of drugs, 6, 123
Strychnine, 21, 145
Sublimation, 73
Substitutes for natural products, 140
Sulfa drugs, 170
Sulfur, 98, 187
Sulphonal, 156, 176
Sumerian drugs, 38
Sunlight, 181
Susrata, 35
Swallowing, 122
Sweating, treatment by, 59
Sweet oil of vitriol (ether), 98, 132
Sympathetic nervous system, 145, 172
Synonymic drug lists, 76, 78
Synonyms of drug names, 77
Synthetic substitute drugs, 141
Syphilis, 95, 171
Syphilis, chemotherapy of, 172
Systema Naturae (Linne's), 111

T

Talmud, 45
Tannin, 19, 120, 177
Taoism, 32
Target organs for drug action, 128, 141
Tea, 105

Temperaments (from humors), 59
Testicular extracts, 175
Tetanus antitoxin, 149
Tetanus toxin, 148
Tetraethyl lead, 185
Thallium salts, 130
Thebaine, 121, 145
Theocratic period of Muslim medicine, 73
Therapeutics, 4
Theriac and Methridatum (Watson), 65
Theriaka of Nicander, 66
Thiamine, 181
Thuja, 113
Thyroid gland, 174
Thyroxine, 174
Time-concentration relations, 6
Time measurement in Sumeria, 39
Tinctures, 73
Toad skins, 34
Toledo, 89
Toxicological studies, 65, 138
Toxicology, 138, 139, 183
Toxicology, definition of, 4
Toxicology, industrial, 184
Trademarked drugs, 159
Traite 'des Poisons (Orfila), 138
Tratado de las Drogues (Acosta), 89
Treacle, 90
Treatise on Poisons (Christison), 138
Treatment by bleeding, purging, vomiting, 59, 131
Tres facies (quatrain of E. Cordus), 91
Tribromethanol, 155
Trochlorethanol, 155
Trional, 156
Trypanosomes, 171
Trypanosomiasis, 172
Trypsin, 182
Tryptamine, 177
Tunis, 73
Typhoid fever, 131

U

Ultra-violet radiation, 181
Undesired drug action, 4
United States Food & Drug Administration, 186

United States Pharmacopeia, 64
University of California, vii, 129
University of Dorpat, 14, 139
University of Edinburgh, 146
University of Pennsylvania, 132, 133
University of Texas, 131
University of Wisconsin, vii, 133
Upas tiente (Borneo arrow poison), 122
Upper Haight-Ashbury (snobbish), viii
Urea, 122, 148, 156
Urea derivatives, 176
Urethane, 156
Uric acid, 122
Utrecht, 151
Uxmal, 41

V

Vaccine for diphtheria, 171
Vaccine standardization, 172
Vagbahata, 35
Vagus nerves, 172
Vasomotor responses, 172
Vehicles for drug administration, 52
Venoms, snake, 115, 146
Veratrine, 120
Veratrum, 63, 120
Verification in natural sciences, 108
Vermifuges, 70
"Veronal," 156
Veterinary treatises, 47, 70
Vikings' "berserksvorgang," 25
Vis medicatrix naturae, 58, 166
Vitamine A, fat-soluble, 181

Vitamin B_1, 180
Vitamin C, 180
Vitamin D, 181
Vitamin E, 182
Vitamin K, 182
Vitamins, 168, 180
Vitriol, 75
Volume measurement, 46
Vomiting, 19, 59, 122
Voyages, Renaissance, 89

W

Water and mineral metabolism, 175
Water balance, 114
whd, Egyptian principle of putrefaction, 51
Willow (Salix), 22, 158, 160
Wine, spirit of, 74
Wines, 23, 85, 86, 90, 129
Wintergreen, oil of, 23, 160
Wisdom of the Body (Cannon), 178
Witch's Sabbath, 28, 100

X

X-rays, 178
X-ray visualization of body cavities, 178

Y

Yaws, 95
Yellow Emperor's Classic (Veith), 31

Z

Zahagun Codices, 53